AF759827

FAMILY, WORK, AND COMMUNITY ISSUES FOR PARENTS OF CHILDREN WITH MENTAL HEALTH DISABILITIES

Family, Work, and Community Issues for Parents of Children with Mental Health Disabilities provides accessible, internationally researched knowledge regarding the challenges of parenting a child with a mental health disability from a social work perspective.

Situating the care of children with mental health disability within a social justice and disability rights framework, it presents current interdisciplinary theories used to examine the phenomena of caring for a child with a mental health disability. Specifically addressing the facilitators and barriers for parents that support or inhibit their ability to manage their exceptional care with other social roles, it provides current international empirical evidence on how parenting a child with a mental health disability affects and is affected by work, family, and community resources. Chapters explore international policy responses to family caregiving of children with mental health disabilities and discuss how the COVID-19 pandemic and its associated shutdowns affected parents of children with mental health disabilities.

This volume will be required reading for social work educators, students, and professionals. It is also relevant for social work practice with children and families, and researchers, teachers, and practitioners in the fields of social policy, public administration, occupational psychology, and disability studies.

Claudia Sellmaier, PhD, MSW, MA, University of Washington Tacoma. With over ten years of experience as a social work researcher and educator, Dr Sellmaier's scholarship centers economic stability and work–life fit in the context of disability with a specific focus on the role of community resources and social policies.

Lisa M. Stewart, PhD, MSW, is a social work scholar and policy expert specializing in family support, children's mental health, and work–family dynamics, with over 18 years of research focused on caregivers of children with mental health needs. Her work bridges research, policy, and practice to develop innovative tools and interventions that support families navigating complex systems at the intersection of health, employment, and social care.

"*Family, Work, and Community Issues for Parents of Children with Mental Health Disabilities: A Guide for Social Workers* provides a careful theoretical and practical analysis of the issues faced by families of children with mental health disabilities, and pathways to develop more substantial workplace and community supports."

Dr. Brennan, *Portland State University, USA*

"Sellmaier and Stewart provide both depth and breadth as they explore the experiences of families caring for children with mental health disorders. Basing the discussion on solid theoretical underpinnings, this book offers a practical perspective on family experiences. This work moves beyond a narrow intra-family view and considers the impact of exceptional caregiving on parent employment and broader community interaction."

Dr. Ana María Brannan, *Indiana University, United States of America*

FAMILY, WORK, AND COMMUNITY ISSUES FOR PARENTS OF CHILDREN WITH MENTAL HEALTH DISABILITIES

A Guide for Social Workers

Claudia Sellmaier and Lisa M. Stewart

Routledge
Taylor & Francis Group
LONDON AND NEW YORK

Designed cover image: Getty Images

First published 2027
by Routledge
4 Park Square, Milton Park, Abingdon, Oxon OX14 4RN

and by Routledge
605 Third Avenue, New York, NY 10158

Routledge is an imprint of the Taylor & Francis Group, an informa business

© 2027 Claudia Sellmaier and Lisa M. Stewart

The right of Claudia Sellmaier and Lisa M. Stewart to be identified as authors of this work has been asserted in accordance with sections 77 and 78 of the Copyright, Designs and Patents Act 1988.

All rights reserved. No part of this book may be reprinted or reproduced or utilised in any form or by any electronic, mechanical, or other means, now known or hereafter invented, including photocopying and recording, or in any information storage or retrieval system, without permission in writing from the publishers.

For Product Safety Concerns and Information please contact our EU representative GPSR@taylorandfrancis.com. Taylor & Francis Verlag GmbH, Kaufingerstraße 24, 80331 München, Germany.

Trademark notice: Product or corporate names may be trademarks or registered trademarks, and are used only for identification and explanation without intent to infringe.

British Library Cataloguing-in-Publication Data
A catalogue record for this book is available from the British Library

ISBN: 978-1-032-87441-8 (hbk)
ISBN: 978-1-032-84737-5 (pbk)
ISBN: 978-1-003-53266-8 (ebk)

DOI: 10.4324/9781003532668

Typeset in Times New Roman
by KnowledgeWorks Global Ltd.

CONTENTS

FIGURES AND TABLES

Figures

Tables

PREFACE

The book *Family, Work, and Community Issues for Parents of Children with Mental Health Disabilities: A Guide for Social Workers* provides an overview of the issues parents encounter when caring for a child with a mental health disability. This book is based on our more than 15 years of research surveying and interviewing parents with exceptional care responsibilities and the research, family support work, and policy advocacy of fellow research and practice colleagues. Families caring for a child with a mental health disability face unique challenges in the workplace, their family systems, and their communities. They are often alone trying to navigate workplace demands and service systems with little financial or instrumental support. Stigmatization exacerbates experiences of stress and isolation. This book aims at providing an overview of both how exceptional care affects work, family, and community systems and how these systems affect families. In addition to discussing families' experiences, the book also includes a discussion of relevant theories to adequately frame and contextualize the empirical evidence. The impact of the Covid-19 pandemic and its longer-term consequences, a comparison of social policies across countries, and a discussion of workplace, therapy, and policy innovations offer insights into the lessons that can be learned from this experience. Each chapter includes recommendations for social work practice and activities that can be used in social work classrooms. Each of the learning activities is connected to the Council of Social Work Education's (CSWE) Educational Policy and Accreditation Standards (EPAS) allowing for an easier transfer into the classroom setting.

Part 1: Definitions and Terminology

We would like to provide initial clarification on terminology used throughout the book. In this book, we use *parent* as a descriptor for caregivers of children with mental health disabilities. We conceptualize *parent* broadly to include biological or adoptive parents, stepparents, kinship caregivers such as grandparents or siblings, and any other friend or relative who provides substantial daily supervision and care for a child with a mental health disability. Furthermore, we use both *person-first and identity-first language* in this book following recommendations by the American Psychological Association. Person-first language uses language such as a person with a disability, while identity-first language would use a description such as a disabled person. Person-first language was adopted to combat stigmatization, but more recently disability activists and different disability groups have advocated for identity-first language (Dunn & Andrews, 2015). Choosing identity-first language can signify autonomy and pride and signals that disability is not considered something wrong but a part of one's identity. Using both person- and identity-first language should represent this discourse and the diverse ways people identify. Respecting human dignity and self-determination guides social work practitioners, and our use of language should be guided by the preferences of the individuals we work with, who might prefer person-first or identity-first language. There will be a more detailed discussion of disability theories in Chapter 2. Finally, we would like to introduce the concept of *exceptional care responsibilities* (Roundtree & Lynch, 2006). Caring for a child with a mental health disability can be considered exceptional care. Exceptional care can be distinguished from typical care in several ways. For example, it is crisis-driven, cyclical, it might not get easier over time, the child might not grow in independence, there might be more interruptions to work and family routines, and the need for navigating health care and educational systems. The family, work, and community issues for parents of children with mental health disabilities discussed in this book therefore fall under the umbrella of exceptional care responsibilities. The chapters in this book will increase the reader's understanding of exceptional care and offer insights into social work practice and advocacy to support this group of parents.

Part 2: Organization of the Book

The book includes ten chapters. The first three chapters provide a theoretical overview and framework that guides the whole approach to the writing. Chapter 1 discusses mental health disabilities in general, Chapter 2 frames exceptional care responsibilities as a social justice issue, and Chapter 3 provides an overview of relevant work and family theories. The second section of the book moves into a description of the experiences of families including a discussion of the effects of exceptional care on the family system (Chapter 4), the interactions of employed parents with the workplace (Chapter 5), and the interactions of families with the community system (Chapter 6). Chapter 7 takes a closer look at work, family, and community issues during the COVID-19 pandemic. In Chapter 8, we conduct a cross-cultural comparison of health care, education, and financial policies. The final chapter in this section discusses innovative trends and new developments (Chapter 9). Chapter 10 summarizes the main themes of exceptional care in the context of work, family, and community systems and discusses future directions in research, practice and advocacy to support parents of children with mental health disabilities. Implications for social work practice and educational activities, which can be used in the classroom, are included at the end of each chapter. A detailed description of each chapter is provided below:

Chapter 1: Understanding Mental Health Disabilities in Children

Part 1 in this chapter discusses the challenges in defining mental health disabilities in children, and part 2 provides international and national prevalence data. Part 3 details the impacts on parenting, followed in part 4 by a discussion of the causes and risk factors for developing a mental health disability. The chapter finishes with a discussion of the importance of early intervention and treatment.

Chapter 2: Exceptional Care as a Social Justice Issue

Chapter 2 frames exceptional care as a social justice issue, discussing in part 1 relevant disability theories followed by a closer examination of disability rights and justice frameworks. Part 3 connects disability theories and disability rights and justice frameworks to exceptional care responsibilities. Finally, the chapter highlights social work ethics and the Grand Challenges of social work and their implications for families caring for a child with a mental health disability.

Chapter 3: The Community, Work, and Family Interface: Theoretical Analysis

Part 1 in Chapter 3 situates exceptional care responsibilities to other life roles, followed by a more detailed discussion of life course, boundaries, and ecological contexts in parenting a child with a mental health disability in part 2. Part 3 highlights theoretical approaches to stigma and family adaptation. The chapter finishes with an exploration of theories related to the continuum of dependent care and work-life fit.

Chapter 4: The Family System

Chapter 4 discusses the effects of exceptional care responsibilities on the family system. Part 1 focuses on the impact on parents as individuals and on their couple's relationship. Part 2 broadens the perspective, discussing the effect on extended family members and friends. In part 3, we take a closer look at the sibling relationship, and we conclude the chapter with a discussion of family resilience in part 4.

Chapter 5: The Work–Family Dilemma

Chapter 5 examines families' interactions with the workplace and their ability to integrate work and family demands. Part 1 discusses work-family integration for families with exceptional care responsibilities. Part 2 highlights the time bind and the complexity of care in these families followed by a discussion of workplace flexibility in part 3. Part 4 examines the challenges to accessing workplace flexibility for parents of children with mental health disabilities. Part 5 takes a closer look at the economic impact of exceptional care, while part 6 discusses the positive impact of employment and work.

Chapter 6: Social Support and Community Resources

Chapter 6 examines the role of social support and community resources for families with exceptional care responsibilities. Part 1 highlights educational policies and programs relevant for children with mental health disabilities. Part 2 focuses on health insurance and mental health care as a possible resource for families. Part 3 discusses peer support and part 4 respite care. Each section describes available policies and programs and barriers to accessing these services.

Chapter 7: The Effects of COVID-19

Chapter 7 considers the effects of the COVID-19 pandemic and its associated shutdowns on families caring for a child with a mental health disability. Part 1 examines the changes to work and community resources followed by a discussion of how these changes affected families in part 2. Part 3 highlights trends and lasting developments beyond the immediate effects of the pandemic.

Chapter 8: Comparative Analysis of Developed Countries' Policies

Chapter 8 introduces a comparative policy analysis framework in part 1. Part 2 moves into the actual comparison between the U.S., Canada, and Germany starting with a discussion of health care policies. Part 3 examines educational policies in these three countries, and part 4 describes financial and leave policies. The final part compares anti-discrimination policies in the United States, Canada, and Germany.

Chapter 9: Emerging Trends and Innovations

Chapter 9 identifies emerging trends and innovations with part 1 focusing on innovations in the workplace. Part 2 introduces innovative family therapeutic approaches, while part 3 discusses new developments in social and workplace policies.

Chapter 10: Summary and Future Directions

Chapter 10 provides a summary and identifies future directions for social work practice, social policy, and social work research.

Part 3: Acknowledgments

We would like to express our gratitude to all the family members who were willing to share their experiences and time with us over the years. This book would not exist without their invaluable insights. We hope that sharing their stories can help change workplaces and communities and can equip social workers with the information and tools to support families, as they navigate work, family, and community systems.

We also want to thank our mentors Drs. Brennan and Rosenzweig for believing in this work and helping us develop the skills to conduct the meaningful research that informs this book. Their enthusiasm kept us going even in challenging times.

Our gratitude also goes to the many colleagues, who joined us on our research path, just to mention Dr. Kim and Dr. Brannan and many more with whom we collaborated or shared critical conversations. We are very lucky to work with so many passionate and brilliant researchers who inspired our work and grew our understanding. We are also thankful to the many MSW students who helped us with our research studies.

We are grateful for the reviewers of the book proposal, our editor Claire Jarvis and all editorial staff from Routledge for their guidance on writing this book.

Finally, we want to thank our families for their encouragement and for believing in us, especially during those long weekend writing sessions. We love you.

References

Dunn, D. S., & Andrews, E. E. (2015). Person-first and identity-first language: Developing psychologists' cultural competence using disability language. *The American Psychologist*, *70*(3), 255–264. https://doi.org/10.1037/a0038636

Roundtree, L., & Lynch, K. (2006). *Exploring the complexities of exceptional caregiving*. Executive briefing series. Boston College, Center for Work & Family.

1

UNDERSTANDING MENTAL HEALTH DISABILITIES IN CHILDREN

Mental health disabilities in children encompass a broad and heterogeneous set of emotional, behavioral, and developmental experiences that affect not only children but also families, schools, health systems, and communities. These conditions are not discrete or static entities. They are shaped by developmental stage, social context, institutional responses, and access to resources (Bronfenbrenner, 1979; National Academies of Sciences, Engineering, and Medicine [NASEM], 2019). As a result, what counts as a mental health disability in childhood often varies across systems and over time, creating uncertainty for families and professionals at the point when concerns first emerge (Bogenschneider, 2024).

A central challenge in this area is the absence of clear boundaries between typical developmental variation and mental health-related impairment. Behaviors such as anxiety, emotional dysregulation, inattention, or withdrawal may be transient, context-specific, or developmentally expected, yet they may also signal emerging mental health needs when persistent and functionally impairing (Baranne & Falissard, 2018; Garralda, 2025). Parents, educators, and practitioners are therefore tasked with interpreting children's behavior under conditions of incomplete information, balancing concerns about over-pathologization with the risks of delayed identification and support (Wakefield & Conrad, 2020).

Definitions of childhood mental health disability are further shaped by the systems families must navigate. Schools, health care providers, insurers, and public agencies rely on different frameworks, terminology, and thresholds for action, often anchored in legal, diagnostic, or administrative requirements rather than lived experience (American Psychiatric Association, 2022; IDEA, 2004). These system-specific definitions determine which children are identified, which services become available, and how prevalence is measured at the population level. As a result, prevalence estimates reflect not only children's mental health needs but also the

DOI: 10.4324/9781003532668-1

structure and priorities of the systems that count them (Whitney & Peterson, 2019). Understanding children's mental health disabilities therefore requires attention not only to symptoms or diagnoses, but also to how meaning is constructed across developmental, institutional, and social contexts. For social workers and allied professionals, this perspective underscores why prevalence data must be interpreted critically and why early encounters with systems can shape family trajectories long before a diagnosis is assigned (Abramovitz & Zelnick, 2022; Gould, 2022).

Part 1: The Challenges in Defining Mental Health Disabilities in Children

Parent, Teacher, and Social Worker Perspectives

Identifying potential mental health disabilities in children is rarely straightforward. As stated in the introduction, parents, educators, social workers, clinicians, and policymakers must interpret children's behavior in contexts where developmental variability, environmental stressors, and institutional expectations overlap. Many behaviors that prompt concern, such as anxiety, tantrums, withdrawal, or difficulty sustaining attention, also fall within the range of typical child development, particularly during periods of transition or stress (Rosenzweig et al., 2008). Distinguishing between developmentally expected variation and emerging mental health need therefore requires judgment under conditions of uncertainty, with meaningful consequences for whether and when children receive support (Baranne & Falissard, 2018; Garralda, 2025).

For parents, this uncertainty is often experienced as a balancing act between fears of over-pathologizing their child and concerns about delaying help when difficulties persist or worsen. Decisions to seek evaluation are shaped not only by the child's behavior but also by access to care, stigma, cost, and the anticipated consequences of labeling across school, health, and insurance systems (Bogenschneider, 2024; Wakefield & Conrad, 2020). These early decisions can shape family trajectories long before any formal diagnosis is assigned.

Educators face parallel challenges. Teachers are frequently among the first to observe emotional or behavioral concerns, yet they operate within classrooms characterized by competing demands, limited training in mental health, and institutional pressures focused on academic performance. Research suggests that while teachers are more likely to recognize severe or externalizing behaviors, they are less likely to identify internalizing problems such as anxiety or depression, which are more easily overlooked and less likely to prompt referral (Deaton et al., 2022; Splett et al., 2019). This pattern has important implications for early identification and helps explain why some children's mental health needs remain invisible until symptoms escalate or academic functioning declines.

Social workers encounter these definitional challenges across diverse practice settings, but do not operate with a single, unified understanding of children's mental health. Instead, social work perspectives are shaped by institutional context, professional role, and theoretical orientation. Table 1.1 summarizes how social workers in school settings often conceptualize mental health in relation to learning, behavior, and peer relationships, focusing on functional barriers to educational participation. Mental health within child welfare contexts is more commonly framed through trauma-informed lenses that emphasize safety, relational disruption, and resilience in the context of adversity (Hoffman et al., 2016). In healthcare and behavioral health settings, clinical social workers are more likely to work within diagnostic frameworks aligned with the DSM-5-TR or ICD-11, where diagnoses structure access to treatment and reimbursement (American Psychiatric Association, 2022; World Health Organization, 2019). Community-based, advocacy, and research-oriented social workers, by contrast, often foreground social determinants of health, racism, immigration status, and structural inequality, resisting narrow diagnostic interpretations in favor of systemic and policy-level analysis (Abramovitz & Zelnick, 2022; Teasley et al., 2022).

Taken together, these perspectives illustrate that children's mental health disabilities are not identified through a single definitional lens. Instead, they are constructed at the intersection of developmental expectations, professional judgment, institutional mandates, and policy rules. This context dependence helps explain why families often receive inconsistent messages across systems and why prevalence estimates vary depending on who is counting, how questions are asked, and which thresholds trigger action (National Academies of Sciences, Engineering, and Medicine [NASEM], 2019; Whitney & Peterson, 2019).

TABLE 1.1 Social Work Practice Setting, Primary Focus, View of Mental Health, and Common Tools or Frameworks for Assessment and Intervention

Practice setting	*Primary focus*	*View of mental health*	*Common tools or frameworks*
School social work	Impact on learning, behavior, and peer relationships	Behavioral or emotional issues interfering with education	Behavioral assessments, IEP teams, RTI
Child welfare	Trauma, safety, and family stability	Outcome of adversity and contributor to family risk	Trauma-informed care, risk assessments
Healthcare/ behavioral health	Clinical symptoms, treatment, and care coordination	Clinical condition requiring treatment and monitoring	DSM-5, ICD-11, treatment plans
Community-based/ advocacy/ research	Social determinants and systemic barriers	Socially influenced condition shaped by inequality and access	Anti-oppressive practice, community organizing

The DSM, Prevalence, and Social Work Critique

Diagnostic frameworks play a central role in shaping how children's mental health needs are recognized, counted, and addressed. In the United States, the Diagnostic and Statistical Manual of Mental Disorders Fifth Edition, Text Revision (DSM-5-TR) functions as the dominant classificatory system across health care, insurance, education-adjacent services, and much of the research literature (American Psychiatric Association [APA], 2022). Although often framed as a technical or clinical tool, the DSM operates as a powerful institutional mechanism that structures access to services, eligibility for accommodations, and the production of population-level prevalence estimates. From a prevalence perspective, DSM-based diagnoses function as gatekeepers. Many national surveys and administrative datasets rely on parent reports of an existing clinical diagnosis or on service utilization that itself requires a DSM-aligned determination. As a result, prevalence estimates frequently reflect differential access to diagnosis rather than the true distribution of mental health need. Children who encounter barriers related to race, socioeconomic status, geography, immigration status, language access, or insurance coverage are less likely to be diagnosed and therefore less likely to be counted (National Academies of Sciences, Engineering, and Medicine [NASEM], 2019; Whitney & Peterson, 2019). In this way, prevalence statistics are shaped as much by institutional pathways into diagnosis as by children's lived experiences of distress or impairment.

The DSM's categorical structure further influences who is rendered visible within prevalence data. Diagnostic thresholds require children to meet specific criteria and demonstrate clinically significant impairment, a process that can be particularly challenging in childhood, where emotional and behavioral expressions are developmentally variable and highly context dependent. Children whose distress is episodic, situational, or closely tied to environmental stressors may fall below diagnostic thresholds despite experiencing meaningful functional impact. These children are often excluded from prevalence counts and may not gain access to services until difficulties escalate (Leeb et al., 2024; Mersky et al., 2021). Consequently, prevalence estimates grounded in DSM diagnoses tend to privilege more severe, persistent, or externally observable presentations, while undercounting internalizing distress and contextually driven suffering.

Social work scholars have long critiqued these dynamics, particularly the medicalization of childhood behavior. Expanding diagnostic categories and increased reliance on psychiatric classification have raised concerns about the pathologization of developmentally normative responses to adversity, stress, and structural inequality. Wakefield's framework has been influential in social work and allied disciplines, highlighting how diagnostic practices may conflate social suffering with disorder when contextual factors are insufficiently considered (Wakefield & Conrad, 2020). From this perspective, diagnosis risks obscuring the social and environmental conditions that produce distress, while redirecting attention toward individual-level treatment rather than structural intervention.

A second major line of critique centers on racialized and culturally patterned diagnosis. Social work scholars, particularly those from marginalized communities, have demonstrated how DSM-based practices contribute to systematic misdiagnosis and differential diagnosis among Black, Latinx, and Indigenous children. Black youth, for example, are more likely to be diagnosed with externalizing or conduct-related disorders and less likely to receive diagnoses associated with internalizing distress, even when presenting with comparable symptoms (Elkins et al., 2019; Thyberg & Lombardi, 2022). These patterns are not simply clinical errors, but outcomes of diagnostic systems that privilege Eurocentric norms of behavior and emotional expression while failing to account for racism, discrimination, and structural trauma (Gray et al., 2013; Lindsey et al., 2013). More recent scholarship situates diagnosis within broader systems of governance, arguing that psychiatric categories function as technologies that regulate marginalized bodies and identities, individualize structural harm, and legitimate surveillance within schools, child welfare, and juvenile justice systems (Pickersgill, 2024).

In response to these concerns, social work scholars increasingly advocate for frameworks that decenter DSM dominance without abandoning assessment altogether. Approaches such as structural competency emphasize the need for practitioners to recognize how policies, institutions, and historical inequities shape presenting concerns, rather than locating distress solely within individual children or families (Gorman Ezell & Stough-Hunter, 2025). Healing-centered engagement similarly reframes mental health around collective well-being, cultural identity, and resistance to oppression, offering an alternative to deficit-oriented diagnostic models (Ginwright, 2018). Indigenous and decolonial scholars further challenge the DSM's universalizing assumptions, emphasizing collective suffering, historical trauma, and culturally grounded healing practices that fall outside Western psychiatric classification systems (Gone & Kirmayer, 2020).

Taken together, these critiques do not reject diagnosis outright but call for a more reflexive and justice-oriented use of diagnostic tools. For social workers, the central task is not to determine whether the DSM is "right" or "wrong," but to understand how diagnostic systems shape visibility, access, and inequity. When prevalence estimates are grounded primarily in DSM-based diagnoses, they must be interpreted as partial and socially produced indicators rather than neutral reflections of children's mental health. A critical social work lens therefore requires asking not only how many children are counted, but who remains unseen, whose distress is legitimized, and how institutional definitions of disorder shape pathways into care.

World Health Organization's Conceptualization of Mental Health Disability

At the global level, the World Health Organization (WHO) conceptualizes children's mental health disability through a population health framework that differs in important ways from DSM-centered approaches dominant in the United States. Rather than privileging individual diagnosis as the primary unit of analysis, the

WHO emphasizes identification, surveillance, and estimation as complementary tools for understanding mental health needs across populations (World Health Organization [WHO], 2014, 2023a). Identification refers to the use of standardized diagnostic criteria, most commonly the ICD-11, to support recognition of mental health conditions within health systems. Surveillance involves the ongoing collection of population-level data to monitor trends, disparities, and service access over time, including among groups who may not be engaged in formal care. Estimation uses statistical modeling to approximate the burden of mental health conditions in contexts where direct data are incomplete or uneven. Together, these approaches are intended to support prevention, equity-focused policy, and system-level planning rather than to determine individual eligibility for services.

This population health orientation stands in contrast to DSM-driven prevalence estimates, which are often anchored to clinical diagnosis and service contact and therefore reflect differential access to care. While DSM-based prevalence tends to privilege children who are visible within health or education systems, WHO estimates are designed to capture broader patterns of need, including unmet need, across countries and contexts. For social workers and policymakers, this distinction matters. WHO-derived prevalence figures are useful for highlighting global burden, cross-national inequities, and the role of social determinants of mental health, but they are less directly tied to individual-level decision-making. Read alongside DSM-based data, the WHO framework underscores that prevalence is not a singular truth but a function of methodological choice, institutional priorities, and the purposes for which data are generated.

Diagnostic Criteria, Diagnosis, and Systemic Barriers in Pediatric Mental Health Care

Diagnostic criteria are intended to promote consistency in identifying mental health conditions, yet in pediatric contexts, they often operate as structural barriers rather than neutral tools. In the United States, access to mental health services across health, education, and insurance systems is frequently contingent on the presence of a formal diagnosis aligned with the DSM-5-TR (American Psychiatric Association [APA], 2022). While diagnosis is positioned as a gateway to care, the pathways to obtaining one are uneven, fragmented, and shaped by institutional constraints that disproportionately affect marginalized families. Across public systems, delays in diagnostic evaluation are common due to workforce shortages, administrative requirements, and restrictive eligibility thresholds. These delays can leave children without support during periods of acute need, particularly when symptoms are complex, comorbid, or do not fit neatly within categorical criteria (Whitney & Peterson, 2019). In private systems, insurance coverage often hinges on diagnostic specificity, resulting in denials of assessment or treatment when children do not meet full criteria, despite clear functional impairment (Houtrow et al., 2025). Together, these dynamics create a system in which diagnosis functions less as a clinical clarification and more as a rationing mechanism. Systemic fragmentation further compounds these barriers.

Educational, medical, and behavioral health systems in the U.S. operate with distinct definitions of need, documentation standards, and thresholds for action. As a result, children may be identified as struggling in one system while remaining ineligible for services in another. Schools may frame concerns in terms of behavior or learning impact without assigning or recognizing clinical diagnoses, while health care providers may delay diagnostic labeling due to stigma concerns or uncertainty about service availability. These misalignments place social workers in the position of translating across systems, often without the authority or resources needed to resolve gaps in care. Importantly, these barriers are not evenly distributed. Diagnostic access is patterned by race, socioeconomic status, language access, geography, and insurance coverage, contributing to persistent disparities in identification and treatment. Children from historically marginalized communities are more likely to experience delayed diagnosis, misdiagnosis, or exclusion from services altogether, reinforcing inequities that are later reflected in prevalence data and long-term outcomes (Elkins et al., 2019; Thyberg & Lombardi, 2022).

Part 2: Prevalence Data (Global and United States)

Purpose and Framing

This section synthesizes global and U.S. prevalence estimates of children's mental health needs to establish scope, trends, and inequities, while avoiding exhaustive cataloging of surveillance systems (Polanczyk et al., 2015; Whitney & Peterson, 2019). Consistent with social work's emphasis on critical use of data, prevalence figures are treated as socially produced indicators shaped by diagnostic frameworks, data collection methods, and policy incentives, rather than as neutral facts.

Global Prevalence: Patterns, and Cautions

Global meta-analyses using standardized diagnostic assessments converge on the conclusion that mental disorders affect a sizable minority of children and adolescents worldwide. Polanczyk and colleagues' pooled estimate across 41 studies in 27 countries suggests that 13.4% of children and adolescents meet criteria for any mental disorder, with pooled estimates of 6.5% for any anxiety disorder, 2.6% for any depressive disorder, 3.4% for attention deficit hyperactivity disorder (ADHD), and 5.7% for any disruptive disorder (Polanczyk et al., 2015). Complementing this disorders-focused evidence, the WHO estimates that about one in seven adolescents ages 10–19, 14%, experience a mental health condition, underscoring both prevalence and burden across the adolescent years (World Health Organization, 2022). Global estimates vary across regions and studies. Differences reflect not only true variation in risk exposure, such as conflict, poverty, displacement, and structural violence, but also methodological factors, including diagnostic criteria, informant sources, functional impairment thresholds, and access to services (Liu et al., 2025;

Polanczyk et al., 2015). International estimates should therefore be interpreted as comparative signals rather than precise counts. From a social work perspective, the most salient contribution of global data is their illumination of inequities and unmet need, particularly in low- and middle-income contexts where service infrastructure and culturally responsive assessment tools remain limited.

U.S. Prevalence: Trends and Inequities

In the United States, national surveillance consistently shows that mental, emotional, and behavioral conditions are common in childhood, with prevalence increasing with age and with meaningful differences by social location. Centers for Disease Control summaries of nationally representative data indicate that nearly 1 in 5 children ages 3–17, about 21%, had ever been diagnosed with a mental, emotional, or behavioral health condition, based on 2021 estimates (Centers for Disease Control and Prevention [CDC], 2025). Using 2022–2023 data, CDC reports current diagnosed prevalence of 11% for anxiety, 8% for behavior disorders, and 4% for depression among children ages 3–17 (Centers for Disease Control and Prevention, 2025). Adolescent-specific estimates underscore the scale of need in secondary school years. A 2023 National Survey of Children's Health brief reports that 20.3% of adolescents ages 12–17 had a current, diagnosed mental or behavioral health condition, anxiety, depression, or behavior or conduct problems, with anxiety at 16.1% and depression at 8.4% (Health Resources and Services Administration, 2024). Prevalence increases across childhood, with adolescence representing a period of heightened identification and service contact. Recent analyses using nationally representative data show that internalizing concerns, particularly anxiety and depressive symptoms, are more frequently identified during early and middle adolescence than in younger childhood, reflecting both developmental processes and increased exposure to academic, social, and economic stressors (Racine et al., 2021; Zablotsky et al., 2023).

The same brief documents increase from 2016 to 2023, including a rise in any current diagnosis from 15.0% to 20.3% (Health Resources and Services Administration, 2024). Contemporary studies suggest that these increases reflect a combination of factors, including expanded screening, greater public and professional awareness, shifts in diagnostic practices, and growing social and economic pressures affecting children and families (Bitsko et al., 2022; Lebrun-Harris et al., 2022). COVID-era research further documents sharp increases in emotional distress among children and adolescents, particularly depressive and anxiety symptoms, highlighting the sensitivity of prevalence patterns to broader social disruption rather than stable underlying pathology alone (Racine et al., 2021). We discuss in depth the implications of COVID on child mental health and implications for parents in a later chapter (Chapter 7).

Three things stand out when examining the prevalence data. First, mental health needs are common and often emerge early in the life course. Second, prevalence estimates are sensitive to diagnostic thresholds and reporting sources, reinforcing critiques of diagnosis-driven frameworks (Wakefield & Conrad, 2020). Third, disparities in identification and treatment mirror broader inequities in education, healthcare, housing, and labor markets, underscoring the necessity of structurally informed intervention and advocacy. Fourth, prevalence is not evenly distributed. Disparities by race and ethnicity, socioeconomic status, insurance coverage, disability status, and geography reflect both heightened recognition and screening and enduring structural barriers that shape who is identified, who receives services, and whose distress is medicalized (World Health Organization, 2022).

Implications for Social Work Education, Practice, and Policy

For social workers, prevalence data function less as definitive measures and more as tools for agenda setting, resource allocation, and systems-level accountability (Gambrill, 2013). Critical engagement with these data requires attention to whose experiences are counted, how categories are defined, and how prevalence statistics are mobilized in policy debates. When paired with ecological and anti-oppressive frameworks, prevalence estimates can support advocacy for prevention, early intervention, culturally responsive services, and family-centered supports that extend beyond diagnosis. From a social work perspective, *assessment literacy*, the ability to understand, question, and contextualize diagnostic and screening practices, is a critical equity issue. Families are frequently asked to engage with assessment results that determine access to services, accommodations, and protections, often without clear explanation of what those results mean, how stable they are, or how they may change over time. For parents, assessment frequently marks an entry point into systems that are difficult to navigate, where labels carry both opportunity and risk. Assessment practices also contribute to *uncertainty* for families over time. Diagnostic categories may shift as children develop, school contexts change, or eligibility criteria are revised. Parents are often required to repeatedly document their child's needs through new assessments to maintain access to services, creating cycles of evaluation that are burdensome, expensive, and destabilizing. In this way, diagnosis functions not as a one-time clarification, but as an ongoing negotiation between families and systems. For social workers, the ethical challenge is not to perfect diagnostic technique, but to critically engage with assessment as a gatekeeping mechanism. This includes recognizing the limits of diagnosis-based prevalence data, advocating for assessments that are culturally responsive and functionally meaningful, and supporting families in interpreting and using assessment information without reinforcing deficit-based narratives. Assessment literacy allows social workers to help families navigate uncertainty while resisting the over-medicalization of distress and the individualization of structural harm.

Thus, diagnosis and assessment are therefore positioned as mechanisms through which prevalence becomes actionable, rather than as neutral reflections of children's mental health status. Understanding how assessment practices shape who is counted, who is served, and who bears the burden of proof is essential for interpreting prevalence data responsibly and for advancing equitable, family-centered systems of care.

BOX 1.1 DIAGNOSIS THROUGH A SOCIAL WORK LENS

When social workers assess children's mental health, they are not simply determining whether diagnostic criteria are met. They are navigating ethical obligations, power dynamics, and structural conditions that shape both symptoms and their interpretation. Competent assessment requires the integration of multiple social work competencies in real time.

Ethical practice and professional judgment are central. Social workers must balance the potential benefits of diagnosis, such as access to services and shared language, against possible harms, including stigma, diagnostic overshadowing, or unintended consequences within schools and other systems (CSWE Competency 1). This often requires transparent conversations with families about how diagnostic information will be used and revisited over time.

Engagement and assessment skills are equally critical. Children's mental health concerns are best understood through multi-informant, multi-context assessment that includes caregivers, educators, and the child, while recognizing that these perspectives may diverge (CSWE Competency 6). Social workers must interpret discrepant reports without defaulting to deficit-based explanations, particularly when behavioral concerns are foregrounded in school settings.

Attention to diversity, equity, and anti-racist practice is essential throughout the assessment process. Historical patterns of over- and under-diagnosis among marginalized children mean that social workers must critically examine how race, culture, language, disability, and socioeconomic conditions influence both symptom expression and professional interpretation (CSWE Competency 2). Cultural humility and awareness of structural inequities are necessary to avoid reinforcing harm through diagnostic decisions.

Assessment also requires systems-level thinking. Social workers routinely operate at the intersection of health care, education, and social services, translating clinical findings into language that supports access to resources without exceeding the limits of diagnosis (CSWE Competencies 4 and 8). This includes recognizing that clinical diagnoses do not determine educational eligibility and advocating for supports based on functional impact rather than labels alone.

Finally, social workers are called to use assessment as a foundation for intervention and ongoing evaluation. Diagnosis should inform, but not constrain, care planning, and should be revisited as children develop and contexts change (CSWE Competency 7). From a social work perspective, effective assessment is an iterative, relational process grounded in ethics, equity, and a commitment to child and family well-being.

Part 3: The Short- and Long-term Impacts of Parenting a Child with a Disability

Over two decades of research on caregiving demands show that the care itself extends well beyond episodic stress, shaping families' economic stability, employment trajectories, physical and mental health, and engagement with service systems over time. These impacts are patterned rather than idiosyncratic, reflecting predictable interactions between caregiving intensity, inadequate formal supports, and institutional arrangements that presume uninterrupted labor force participation and individual responsibility for care (U.S. Department of Health and Human Services, 2021). From a life-course perspective, the consequences of caregiving are cumulative. Employment disruptions, reduced earnings, and increased out-of-pocket costs compound across developmental stages, particularly when children's needs intensify during school transitions or adolescence. Caregiver stress and psychological distress are therefore best understood not as individual coping failures but as outcomes of sustained exposure to structural strain, including underinsurance, fragmented service systems, and limited workplace flexibility (Brown & Clark, 2017; Validova et al., 2023). For parents, these cumulative impacts are experienced not as discrete stressors but as ongoing navigation through uncertain systems of care, employment, and education, in which eligibility, expectations, and supports shift across developmental stages.

Importantly, the impacts documented are unevenly distributed. Families marginalized by race, ethnicity, immigration status, income, and geography experience heightened exposure to both caregiving demands and systemic barriers to support. These inequities mirror broader patterns in mental health identification and service access discussed earlier in the chapter, reinforcing the need for anti-oppressive and structurally responsive approaches to family support.

Exceptional Caregiving as a Long-term Social Problem

Exceptional caregiving refers to caregiving responsibilities that exceed normative, developmentally expected family care due to the intensity, unpredictability, and duration of disability- or mental health–related needs, requiring sustained coordination, specialized knowledge, and ongoing resource negotiation across the life course (Roundtree & Lynch, 2006; Stewart et al., 2022). Exceptional caregiving, particularly when it involves caring for a child with a mental health disability like depression or obsessive compulsive behavior (OCD), autism spectrum disorder (ASD), ADHD, or serious emotional disturbance, is best understood as a long-term social condition rather than a transient family challenge. Unlike normative parenting demands, which generally decline as children age, mental health-related caregiving often persists across developmental stages, intensifies during periods of crisis, and, in many cases, extends into adulthood. This extended time horizon fundamentally alters parents' relationships to work, health, and social institutions, producing cumulative consequences that exceed what individual families can reasonably absorb.

Longitudinal research has been especially important in documenting these long-term effects. Seltzer et al. (2001) work with aging parents of adults with serious mental illness demonstrates that parenting under conditions of chronic psychiatric disability carries enduring psychological and physiological costs well into later life. Using daily diary and biomarker data, Barker et al. (2012) found that parents of adults with serious mental illness exhibited altered diurnal cortisol patterns following high-stress days, a profile consistent with long-term stress-related dysregulation. These findings provide rare biological evidence that decades of caregiving exposure can "get under the skin," shaping parents' health trajectories long after their children reach adulthood. Importantly, this body of work reframes parenting as an open-ended caregiving role, challenging assumptions that parental burden resolves as children age.

Population-based studies further demonstrate that these impacts are not confined to rare or extreme cases. Using nationally representative U.S. data, Witt and colleagues showed that parents of children with activity-limiting conditions, including mental and behavioral health needs, experience significantly poorer physical and mental health and higher rates of work loss than parents of children without such limitations (Witt et al., 2009). Subsequent analyses reinforced these findings, highlighting how child mental health needs interact with socioeconomic status and family structure to shape parental health and employment outcomes over time (Garbarski & Witt, 2013). Together, these studies establish that the health effects of exceptional caregiving are not merely emotional or subjective, but observable at the population level and closely tied to labor market participation.

Research on ASD and ADHD further underscores the chronic nature of caregiving-related strain. Longitudinal and meta-analytic studies consistently document elevated parenting stress, disrupted family functioning, and sustained caregiving demands among parents of children with ASD and ADHD, particularly when behavioral challenges persist across developmental stages (Theule et al., 2013). Emerging physiological research suggests that chronic stress exposure among these parents may be reflected in altered cortisol regulation, reinforcing concerns about long-term health consequences rather than short-term adjustment difficulties.

Critically, U.S. policy structures remain poorly aligned with the realities of long-term mental health caregiving. Employment-based health insurance, limited paid leave, and fragmented mental health service systems place the burden of managing chronic care squarely on families. As Heymann and colleagues have shown, inadequate workplace protections and lack of caregiving supports are associated with poorer health outcomes among employed caregivers, highlighting how policy environments can either mitigate or amplify caregiving-related harm (Earle & Heymann, 2011). Taken together, this evidence supports framing exceptional caregiving as a social problem rooted in the intersection of chronic mental health needs, labor market structures, and policy gaps. The long-term health, economic, and social consequences experienced by parents are not the result of individual vulnerability or poor coping, but of sustained exposure to caregiving demands in systems that provide limited accommodation or protection. Recognizing exceptional caregiving as a long-duration social condition is essential for understanding why work, health, and policy must be addressed together, a theme that anchors the chapters that follow.

Implications for Social Work Practice and Policy

For social workers, evidence from the research base on caregiving points to the necessity of moving beyond child-focused intervention alone. Effective practice requires attending to caregiver well-being, employment conditions, and material hardship as integral components of children's mental health support. At the policy level, these findings strengthen the case for paid family leave, income supports, accessible behavioral health services, and workplace accommodations that recognize caregiving as a sustained social role rather than a temporary disruption. We will discuss the intersection of exceptional care and family systems in Chapter 4, work in Chapter 5, and community systems in Chapter 6.

BOX 1.2 FAMILY IMPACTS OF CHILDREN'S MENTAL HEALTH CONDITIONS

Economic. *Families of children with mental health disabilities are more likely to face financial hardship, problems paying medical bills, and delayed or forgo care, so insurance adequacy and cost protections directly affect family stability (Houtrow et al., 2025; Validova et al., 2023).*

Work. *Caregiving demands frequently lead parents to cut hours or leave jobs, especially with greater symptom severity, so flexible, family-supportive workplace policies help sustain employment (Foster et al., 2021; Sellmaier et al., 2020; Stewart et al., 2023).*

Social. *Families report lower neighborhood support and more access barriers, with rural families often more affected, so reliable school and community services are essential to reduce isolation and strain (Cree et al., 2018; Robinson et al., 2017).*

Caregiver health. *Parents of children with mental or behavioral difficulties report worse mental health and elevated stress, which improves when workplaces and community systems are supportive* (Stewart et al., 2023; Wolicki et al., 2021).

Part 4: Causes and Risk Factors Associated with Mental Health Disabilities in Children

Mental health disabilities in childhood arise from multiple, interacting influences that unfold across development. Contemporary models emphasize an interplay of many genes with experiences in the child's environments, home, school, peers, neighborhoods, and with neurobiological systems that are particularly plastic in early life and adolescence. Large genomics studies show that common psychiatric conditions (e.g., ADHD, autism, depression) are highly polygenic: many variants of small effect contribute to risk, and rare genetic variants can also play a role; at the same time, the field has moved past single "candidate gene" explanations that failed to replicate (Border et al., 2019; Grove et al., 2019; Howard et al., 2019).

On the environmental side, adverse childhood experiences (ACEs), including abuse, neglect, and household challenges, show graded associations with later mental, behavioral, and physical health and have been found to be preventable through policies that strengthen safe, stable, nurturing relationships and environments (; Centers for Disease Control and Prevention, 2024; Hughes et al., 2017; Merrick et al., 2018). Exposure to toxicants (e.g., lead) and air pollution has been linked in systematic reviews to elevated risks of ADHD and depressive symptoms, respectively, underscoring the role of the built environment in neurodevelopment (Dimitrov et al., 2024). Neurobiological research connects early adversity with alterations in stress-response and emotion-regulation circuitry (amygdala–prefrontal networks) and in the hypothalamic–pituitary–adrenal (HPA) axis, helping to explain how experiences "get under the skin" to affect cognition, affect, and behavior and have a "*cumulative effect*" on mental health (Coleman & Stewart, 2010; McLaughlin et al., 2014; Teicher et al., 2016). Last, parenting practices (warmth, autonomy support, consistent behavioral control) have been found to be modestly protective, whereas harsh or psychologically controlling styles and high interparental conflict are associated with higher internalizing and externalizing symptoms (Pinquart, 2017; van Eldik et al., 2020).

Finally, broader social determinants, poverty, material hardship, and neighborhood disadvantage, elevate risk and often co-occur with other stressors, suggesting that effective prevention spans policy, community, school, family, and clinical levers (National Academies of Sciences, Engineering, and Medicine [NASEM], 2019).

BOX 1.3 WHAT ASSESSMENT SCORES CAN AND CANNOT TELL YOU

Assessment scores are often treated as definitive answers, but they are better understood as signals that guide further inquiry.

What scores can tell you

- *Whether a child's reported symptoms are elevated relative to age-based norms*
- *Which domains, such as attention, mood, anxiety, or behavior, warrant closer assessment*
- *Whether symptoms appear to be changing over time or in response to intervention*

What scores cannot tell you

- *Why symptoms are occurring*
- *Whether distress reflects trauma exposure, neurodevelopmental differences, learning demands, or environmental stress*
- *What services a child should receive in isolation from functional and contextual information*

Why this matters

Most standardized tools are designed to identify risk, not to establish diagnosis or predict outcomes. Treating cut scores as final determinations can reinforce inequities, particularly for children who face barriers to comprehensive evaluation or whose behavior is more likely to be interpreted as problematic rather than contextual.

Common misrepresentations social workers are asked to correct

In practice, social workers are frequently asked to explain or reconcile assessment results that have already been interpreted by others. Common misinterpretations include:

- *Assuming that a positive screener is equivalent to a diagnosis*
- *Treating one informant's report, often a school report, as inherently more valid than caregiver or youth perspectives*
- *Interpreting disruptive or externalizing behavior without assessing anxiety, trauma, sleep, or learning demands*
- *Using scores to justify exclusion from services rather than access to support*

Correcting these misinterpretations is a core component of ethical practice and advocacy, especially when assessment results carry consequences across health, education, or legal systems.

How assessment tools shape system decisions

Assessment tools do not operate neutrally. Their results are routinely used to trigger decisions across systems:

- ***Healthcare**: insurance authorization, service intensity, medication approval*
- ***Education**: eligibility for evaluation, accommodations, or special education supports*
- ***Child welfare and juvenile systems**: risk framing, service thresholds, and supervision decisions*

Because these decisions can alter children's trajectories, social workers have a responsibility to contextualize scores, document functioning clearly, and resist pressure to use assessment tools as gatekeeping mechanisms rather than as supports.

An equity lens on assessment

Standardized tools are only as equitable as their interpretation. Equity-informed assessment requires ongoing attention to:

- *Language access, literacy, and cultural meaning-making*
- *Differential exposure to trauma, poverty, racism, and surveillance*
- *Historic patterns of over- and under-diagnosis among Black, Indigenous, and other marginalized children*
- *The mismatch between standardized norms and lived contexts*

Embedding an equity lens does not require abandoning standardized tools, but it does require refusing to treat them as neutral or complete representations of children's experiences.

Taken together, these tools and interpretive practices reinforce a central theme of this chapter: how mental health difficulties are measured shapes what is seen, what is counted, and who receives support. *Just as prevalence estimates depend on survey design and access to diagnosis, assessment results depend on who is asked, which tools are used, and how scores are interpreted within systems.*

Part 5: Early Intervention as a Site of Uncertainty and Uneven Access

In contemporary social work policy and practice discourse, early intervention is frequently positioned as a solution to rising prevalence of children's mental health needs. Recent population-level research continues to support the potential benefits of timely, developmentally appropriate supports, particularly when interventions are embedded in everyday settings such as schools, primary care, and early childhood systems (Fusar-Poli et al., 2022; Radez et al., 2021). However, within a chapter focused on prevalence and uncertainty, early intervention is best understood not as a uniform response, but as a system characterized by uneven access, shifting eligibility criteria, and substantial variation in implementation.

For families, early intervention often becomes a point at which uncertainty intensifies rather than resolves. Recent U.S. studies document persistent gaps between identified mental health needs and receipt of early services, with disparities by race and ethnicity, insurance status, geography, and disability status remaining pronounced (Lebrun-Harris et al., 2022; Zablotsky et al., 2023). COVID-era research further illustrates how disruptions to schools, healthcare, and community services widened these gaps, particularly for children requiring early supports that depend on in-person identification and referral pathways (Racine et al., 2021; Samji et al., 2022). As a result, early intervention frequently functions as a gatekeeping system that parents must navigate under conditions of limited information and constrained choice.

Prevalence data are increasingly used to justify investments in early intervention infrastructure, yet recent scholarship cautions that identification alone does not guarantee timely or equitable access to services. Structural factors, including workforce shortages, fragmented funding streams, and reliance on diagnosis-based eligibility, continue to shape who benefits from early intervention and who remains underserved (Braveman et al., 2022; Kazdin & Blase, 2011). In this chapter, early intervention is therefore positioned as part of the broader landscape parents encounter following identification, one that transforms prevalence statistics into lived experiences of waiting, advocacy, and uncertainty. A fuller examination of early intervention models, effectiveness, and implementation appears in a later chapter.

Part 6: Summary and Key Points

This chapter examined children's mental health prevalence through a population health and social work lens, emphasizing that what is known about children's mental health is shaped by how concerns are defined, measured, and operationalized across systems. Drawing on national and international data, the chapter demonstrated that mental health needs among children and youth are widespread, but that prevalence estimates vary substantially depending on whether they are based on symptoms, diagnoses, service use, or administrative records. These variations are consequential because access to assessment and services is uneven and patterned by race, socioeconomic status, geography, disability, and system involvement. Consistent with social work's commitment to ethical and reflective practice, the chapter traced how diagnostic frameworks, assessment practices, and population surveillance interact to determine who is counted and who remains invisible. Diagnosis was positioned as a tool for communication and access rather than a definitive account of need, underscoring the importance of critical interpretation, attention to functional impairment and developmental context, and awareness of the potential harms of diagnosis-driven approaches, particularly for marginalized children and families. The chapter also engaged the competency of diversity and difference by centering how structural inequities shape identification, service eligibility, and caregiving burden. Through applied case material, parents' experiences of navigating uncertainty were highlighted to illustrate how families make decisions under conditions of incomplete information, financial strain, and social risk. Caregiver hesitation was reframed as active navigation of complex systems, reinforcing the need for social workers to engage families with humility, transparency, and responsiveness. Finally, the chapter emphasized the use of research-informed practice to advance human rights and social, economic, and environmental justice. By underscoring that prevalence and assessment are not neutral exercises but mechanisms that shape pathways into care, the chapter framed children's mental health as a family, systems, and equity issue that unfolds across development, setting the foundation for ethically grounded intervention, advocacy, and policy engagement in the chapters that follow.

Part 7: Application for Social Work Education

Competency 2: Advance Human Rights and Social, Racial, Economic, and Environmental Justice
Competency 3: Engage Anti-Racism, Diversity, Equity, and Inclusion (ADEI) in Practice
Competency 7: Assess Individuals, Families, Groups, Organizations, and Communities
Competency 8: Intervene with Individuals, Families, Groups, Organizations, and Communities

APPLIED CASE STUDY: NAVIGATING IDENTIFICATION, DIAGNOSIS, AND SUPPORT

Maria and James are parents of a nine-year-old child, Lucas, who has recently begun experiencing escalating emotional and behavioral difficulties at school and at home. Teachers report increased irritability, difficulty concentrating, and frequent visits to the school counselor. At home, Lucas exhibits sleep disruption and heightened anxiety, particularly around school mornings. While these concerns have emerged gradually, recent school communications prompt the family to seek guidance.

As Maria and James begin navigating possible explanations and next steps, they encounter a familiar but disorienting terrain. Initial conversations focus on whether Lucas's behavior reflects a transient developmental phase, a response to environmental stressors, or an emerging mental health condition. Each interpretation carries different implications for assessment, disclosure, and access to support. The family's uncertainty is compounded by inconsistent messaging across school staff, pediatric providers, and informal social networks.

Following a school-based screening, Maria and James are advised to pursue a formal evaluation to determine eligibility for accommodations or services. This recommendation introduces a series of decisions that are framed as procedural but experienced as consequential. The family must decide whether to consent to further assessment, how to interpret preliminary findings, and whether a diagnosis might provide access to needed supports or introduce stigma and long-term labeling. These decisions are made under time pressure and with limited clarity about how assessment results will be used across systems.

As the process unfolds, the family encounters variability in thresholds and expectations. The pediatric provider emphasizes symptom monitoring and suggests a wait-and-see approach, while the school underscores documentation requirements tied to service eligibility. Insurance coverage limits assessment options, and waitlists delay follow-up. Throughout this period, Maria and James are asked to repeatedly recount Lucas's challenges, translate between professional languages, and advocate for coherence across systems that operate with different mandates and timelines.

Importantly, the family's navigation does not follow a linear path. As Lucas's needs shift, so do the interpretations of his behavior and the relevance of prior assessments. Recommendations evolve, diagnoses are discussed and reconsidered, and the family must continually recalibrate their understanding of what support is appropriate and attainable. What began as concern about school performance becomes an ongoing negotiation of identity, need, and responsibility.

What to Notice

This case illustrates how prevalence, diagnosis, and intervention converge in families' everyday experiences. First, population-level prevalence data shape when concerns are taken seriously and which pathways become available, yet these data are encountered by families indirectly, through screening tools, eligibility criteria, and professional judgment. Second, assessment functions as both an access point and a gatekeeping mechanism, generating uncertainty rather than resolution as families move across systems with differing thresholds and incentives. Third, parental decision-making is not a single event, but an iterative process shaped by shifting information, institutional constraints, and concern for a child's well-being over time.

From a social work perspective, the case underscores the importance of supporting families not only through discrete decisions, but through sustained navigation under conditions of uncertainty. It highlights the ethical imperative to promote assessment literacy, to contextualize diagnostic information, and to advocate for systems that reduce rather than reproduce fragmentation and inequity. Most importantly, it centers parents as active agents who must make sense of prevalence statistics, causal narratives, and service structures while caring for a child whose needs are still unfolding.

Discussion Questions: Resources, Navigation, and the Applied Case

1. In the applied case, which resources are visible to the parents early on, and which remain hidden or difficult to access? How does this reflect broader patterns in how systems translate prevalence into support?
2. How might the availability of multiple assessments, frameworks, and recommendations contribute to confusion rather than clarity for families like Maria and James? What role can social workers play in supporting assessment literacy without overwhelming parents?

3 Which resources in the case appear to function as gateways to support, and which operate as barriers? How do eligibility rules and documentation requirements shape the family's navigation experience?
4 How might the family's experience of locating and using resources differ if they faced additional barriers related to race, language, immigration status, income, or geography? Which resource categories are most sensitive to these inequities?
5 What informal or peer-based resources might support this family alongside formal systems? How do these resources complement or compensate for gaps in institutional support?
6 At what points in the case could a social worker intervene to help the family identify, interpret, or prioritize resources? How might this differ from simply providing a list of services?
7 How do resource needs change as the child's situation evolves? What does this suggest about the limits of one-time referrals or static resource lists?

Resource List

This chapter draws on a wide range of diagnostic tools, population datasets, and conceptual frameworks that shape how children's mental health needs are identified, measured, and addressed. The resources below are provided to support assessment literacy, data interpretation, teaching, and family navigation. Inclusion does not imply endorsement of any single framework or tool in isolation.

Recommended Books

Brennan, E. M., & Rosenzweig, J. M. (Eds.) (2008). Work, life, and the mental health system of care: A guide for professionals supporting families of children with emotional or behavioral disorders. Paul H. Brookes.
Turner, F. J. (Ed.) (2017). Social work treatment: Interlocking theoretical approaches (6th ed.). Oxford University Press.
Walsh, J. (2015). Clinical assessment in social work: A guide to the biopsychosocial approach (2nd ed.). Lyceum Books.

How to Use These Resources

These tools and datasets are most useful when read in context. Diagnostic instruments support identification and monitoring, not standalone conclusions. Population surveys and administrative data illuminate patterns and inequities, not individual need. Together, these resources can help social workers, allied professionals, students, and parents interpret children's mental health information critically, advocate effectively, and navigate systems with greater clarity.

References

Abramovitz, M., & Zelnick, J. R. (2022). Structural racism, managerialism, and the future of the human services: Rewriting the rules. *Social Work*, *67*(1), 8–16. https://doi.org/10.1093/sw/swab051

American Psychiatric Association (2013). *Diagnostic and statistical manual of mental disorders* (5th ed.). https://doi.org/10.1176/appi.books.9780890425596

American Psychiatric Association (2022). *Diagnostic and statistical manual of mental disorders* (5th ed., text rev.). https://doi.org/10.1176/appi.books.9780890425787

Baranne, M. L., & Falissard, B. (2018). Global burden of mental disorders among children aged 5–14 years. *Child and Adolescent Psychiatry and Mental Health*, *12*(1), 19. https://doi.org/10.1186/s13034-018-0225-4

Barker, E. T., Greenberg, J. S., Seltzer, M. M., & Almeida, D. M. (2012). Daily stress and cortisol patterns in parents of adult children with serious mental illness. *Health Psychology*, *31*(1), 130–134. https://doi.org/10.1037/a0025325

Bitsko, R. H., Claussen, A. H., & Lichstein, J., et al. (2022). Mental health surveillance among children—United States, 2013–2019. *MMWR Supplements*, *71*. https://doi.org/10.15585/mmwr.su7102a1

Bogenschneider, K. (2024). Why we should focus on families in policymaking, and why we don't. In *Family policy matters: How policymaking affects families and what professionals can do* (4th ed.). London: Routledge.

Border, R., Johnson, E. C., Evans, L. M., Smolen, A., Berley, N., Sullivan, P. F., & Keller, M. C. (2019). No support for historical candidate gene or candidate gene-by-interaction hypotheses for major depression across multiple large samples. *American Journal of Psychiatry*, *176*(5), 376–387. https://doi.org/10.1176/appi.ajp.2018.18070881

Braveman, P. A., Arkin, E., Proctor, D., Kauh, T., & Holm, N. (2022). Systemic and structural racism: Definitions, examples, health damages, and approaches to dismantling. *Health Affairs*, *41*(2), 171–178. https://doi.org/10.1377/hlthaff.2021.01394

Bronfenbrenner, U. (1979). *The ecology of human development: Experiments by nature and design*. Harvard University Press.

Brown, T. J., & Clark, C. (2017). Employed parents of children with disabilities and work family life balance: A literature review. *Child & Youth Care Forum*, *46*(6), 857–876. https://doi.org/10.1007/s10566-017-9407-0

Centers for Disease Control and Prevention (2024). 2023 Youth Risk Behavior Survey results. https://www.cdc.gov/yrbs/results/2023-yrbs-results.html

Centers for Disease Control and Prevention (2025). Data and statistics on children's mental health. https://www.cdc.gov/children-mental-health/data-research/index.html

Centers for Disease Control and Prevention (2025). CDC WONDER: Online databases and suicide data and statistics. https://wonder.cdc.gov/

Child and Adolescent Health Measurement Initiative (2026). About the National Survey of Children's Health. https://www.childhealthdata.org/learn-about-the-nsch/NSCH

Coleman, D., & Stewart, L. M. (2010). Prevalence and impact of childhood maltreatment in incarcerated youth. *The American Journal of Orthopsychiatry*, *80*(3), 343–349. https://doi.org/10.1111/j.1939-0025.2010.01038.x

Cree, R. A., Bitsko, R. H., Robinson, L. R., Holbrook, J. R., Danielson, M. L., Smith, C., … Bethell, C. (2018). Health care, family, and community factors associated with mental, behavioral, and developmental disorders and poverty among children aged 2–8 years, United States, 2016. *MMWR. Morbidity and Mortality Weekly Report*, *67*(50), 1377–1383. https://doi.org/10.15585/mmwr.mm6750a1

Deaton, J. D., Ohrt, J. H., Linich, K., Wymer, B., Toomey, M., Lewis, O., Guest, J. D., & Newton, T. (2022). Teachers' experiences with K-12 students' mental health. *Psychology in the Schools*, *59*, 932–949. https://doi.org/10.1002/pits.22658

Dimitrov, L. V., Kaminski, J. W., Holbrook, J. R., Bitsko, R. H., Yeh, M., Courtney, J. G., O'Masta, B., Maher, B., Cerles, A., McGowan, K., & Rush, M. (2024). A systematic review and meta-analysis of chemical exposures and Attention-Deficit/Hyperactivity Disorder in children. *Prevention Science: The Official Journal of the Society for Prevention Research*, *25*(Suppl 2), 225–248. https://doi.org/10.1007/s11121-023-01601-6

Earle, A., & Heymann, J. (2011). Protecting the health of employees caring for family members with special health care needs. *Social Science & Medicine*, *73*(1), 68–78. https://doi.org/10.1016/j.socscimed.2011.05.016

Elkins, J., Briggs, H.E., Miller, K.M. (2019). Racial/ethnic differences in the impact of Adverse Childhood Experiences on Posttraumatic Stress Disorder in a nationally representative sample of adolescents. *Child & Adolescent Social Work Journal*, *36*, 449–457. https://doi.org/10.1007/s10560-018-0585-x

Foster, C. C., Chorniy, A., Kwon, S., Kan, K., Heard-Garris, N., & Davis, M. M. (2021). Children with special health care needs and forgone family employment. *Pediatrics*, *148*(3), e2020035378. https://doi.org/10.1542/peds.2020-035378

Fusar-Poli, P., Manchia, M., Koutsouleris, N., Leslie, D., Woopen, C., Calkins, M. E., Dunn, M., Tourneau, C. L., Mannikko, M., Mollema, T., Oliver, D., Rietschel, M., Reininghaus, E. Z., Squassina, A., Valmaggia, L., Kessing, L. V., Vieta, E., Correll, C. U., Arango, C., & Andreassen, O. A. (2022). Ethical considerations for precision psychiatry: A roadmap for research and clinical practice. *European Neuropsychopharmacology*, *63*, 17–34. https://doi.org/10.1016/j.euroneuro.2022.08.001

Gambrill, E. (2013). *Critical thinking in clinical practice: Improving the accuracy of judgments and decisions* (3rd ed.). Oxford University Press.

Garbarski, D., & Witt, W. P. (2013). Child health, maternal marital and socioeconomic factors, and maternal health. *Journal of Family Issues*, *34*(4), 484–509. https://doi.org/10.1177/0192513X12443052

Garralda,M. E. (2025). Child and adolescent psychiatric disorders and ICD-11. *The British Journal of Psychiatry: The Journal of Mental Science*, *226*(4), 200–202. https://doi.org/10.1192/bjp.2024.200

Ginwright, S. (2018). *The future of healing: Shifting from trauma-informed care to healing-centered engagement* [PDF]. https://www.hsredesign.org/wp-content/uploads/2019/03/The-Future-of-Healing-Shifting-From-Trauma-Informed-Care-to-Healing-Centered-En.pdf

Gone, J. P., & Kirmayer, L. J. (2020). Advancing Indigenous mental health research: Ethical, conceptual, and methodological challenges. *Transcultural Psychiatry*, *57*(2), 235–249. https://doi.org/10.1177/1363461520923151

Gorman Ezell, K., & Stough-Hunter, A. (2025). The need for adoption of a structural competency framework in social work education. *Health & Social Work*, *50*(2), 153–156. https://doi.org/10.1093/hsw/hlaf009

Gould, N. (2022). The social work role in mental health services. In *Mental health social work in context* (3rd ed., pp. 46–65). Routledge. https://doi.org/10.4324/9781003181323

Gray, M., Coates, J., & Yellow Bird, M. (Eds.). (2013). *Decolonizing social work*. Routledge. https://doi.org/10.4324/9781315576206

Grove, J., Ripke, S., Als, T. D., Mattheisen, M., Walters, R. K., Won, H., … Børglum, A. D. (2019). Identification of common genetic risk variants for autism spectrum disorder. *Nature Genetics*, *51*(3), 431–444. https://doi.org/10.1038/s41588-019-0344-8

Health Resources and Services Administration, Maternal and Child Health Bureau. (2024). National Survey of Children's Health: Adolescent mental and behavioral health, 2023 [Data brief]. https://mchb.hrsa.gov/sites/default/files/mchb/data-research/nsch-data-brief-adolescent-mental-behavioral-health-2023.pdf

Health Resources and Services Administration, Maternal and Child Health Bureau. (2026). National Survey of Children's Health (NSCH). https://mchb.hrsa.gov/data-research/national-survey-childrens-health

Hoffmann, J. A., Alegría, M., Alvarez, K., Anosike, A., Shah, P. P., Simon, K. M., & Lee, L. K. (2022). Disparities in pediatric mental and behavioral health conditions: A state-of-the-art review. *Pediatrics*, *150*(4), e2022058227. https://doi.org/10.1542/peds.2022-058227

Houtrow, A. J., Shearer, C. S., McKernan, G., Kuhlthau, K., & Agrawal, R. (2025). Health care cost concerns and hardships for families of children with disabilities. *JAMA Network Open*, *8*(4), e257826. https://doi.org/10.1001/jamanetworkopen.2025.7826

Howard, D. M., Adams, M. J., Clarke, T. K., Hafferty, J. D., Gibson, J., Shirali, M., Coleman, J. R. I., Hagenaars, S. P., Ward, J., Wigmore, E. M., Alloza, C., Shen, X., Barbu, M. C., Xu, E. Y., Whalley, H. C., Marioni, R. E., Porteous, D. J., Davies, G., Deary, I. J., Hemani, G., … McIntosh, A. M. (2019). Genome-wide meta-analysis of depression identifies 102 independent variants and highlights the importance of the prefrontal brain regions. *Nature Neuroscience*, *22*(3), 343–352. https://doi.org/10.1038/s41593-018-0326-7

Hughes, K., Bellis, M. A., Hardcastle, K. A., Sethi, D., Butchart, A., Mikton, C., Jones, L., & Dunne, M. P. (2017). The effect of multiple adverse childhood experiences on health: A systematic review and meta-analysis. *The Lancet. Public Health*, *2*(8), e356–e366. https://doi.org/10.1016/S2468-2667(17)30118-4

Individuals with Disabilities Education Improvement Act of 2004, 20 U.S.C. § 1400 (2004).

Institute for Health Metrics and Evaluation (2020). GBD 2019 disease and injury burden 1990–2019. Global Health Data Exchange. https://ghdx.healthdata.org/record/ihme-data/gbd-2019-disease-and-injury-burden-1990-2019

Kazdin, A. E., & Blase, S. L. (2011). Interventions and models of their delivery to reduce the burden of mental illness: Reply to commentaries. *Perspectives on Psychological Science*, *6*(5), 507–510. https://doi.org/10.1177/1745691611418241

Lebrun-Harris, L. A., Ghandour, R. M., Kogan, M. D., & Warren, M. D. (2022). Five-year trends in US children's health and well-being, 2016–2020. *JAMA Pediatrics*, *176*(7), e220056. https://doi.org/10.1001/jamapediatrics.2022.0056

Leeb, R. T., Danielson, M. L., Claussen, A. H., Robinson, L. R., Lebrun-Harris, L. A., & Ghandour, R. et al (2024). Trends in mental, behavioral, and developmental disorders among children and adolescents in the United States, 2016–2021. *Preventing Chronic Disease*, *21*, Article 240142. http://dx.doi.org/10.5888/pcd21.240142

Lindsey, M. A., Chambers, K., Pohle, C., Beall, P., & Lucksted, A. (2013). Understanding the behavioral determinants of mental health service use by urban, under-resourced black youth: Adolescent and caregiver perspectives. *Journal of Child and Family Studies*, *22*(1), 107–121. https://doi.org/10.1007/s10826-012-9668-z

Liu, Z., Liu, Y., Yan, L., & Li, Q. (2025). Trends in the global burden of disease for mental disorders among children aged 0-14 years, 1990-2021. *Journal of Affective Disorders*, *385*, 119325. https://doi.org/10.1016/j.jad.2025.04.156

McLaughlin, K. A., Sheridan, M. A., & Lambert, H. K. (2014). Childhood adversity and neural development: Deprivation and threat as distinct dimensions of early experience. *Neuroscience & Biobehavioral Reviews*, *47*, 578–591. https://doi.org/10.1016/j.neubiorev.2014.10.012

Merrick, M. T., Ford, D. C., Ports, K. A., & Guinn, A. S. (2018). Prevalence of adverse childhood experiences from the 2011-2014 behavioral risk factor surveillance system in 23 States. *JAMA Pediatrics*, *172*(11), 1038–1044. https://doi.org/10.1001/jamapediatrics.2018.2537

Mersky, J. P., Choi, C., Plummer Lee, C., & Janczewski, C. E. (2021). Disparities in adverse childhood experiences by race/ethnicity, gender, and economic status: Intersectional analysis of a nationally representative sample. *Child Abuse & Neglect*, *117*, 105066. https://doi.org/10.1016/j.chiabu.2021.105066

National Academies of Sciences, Engineering, and Medicine (2019). *Fostering healthy mental, emotional, and behavioral development in children and youth: A national agenda.* The National Academies Press. https://doi.org/10.17226/25201

Pickersgill, M. (2024). Stalling or oiling the engines of diagnosis? Shifting perspectives on the DSM and categorical diagnosis in psychiatry. *Sociology of Health & Illness*, *46*(S1), 132–151. https://doi.org/10.1111/1467-9566.13682

Pinquart, M. (2017). Associations of parenting dimensions and styles with internalizing symptoms in children and adolescents: A meta-analysis. *Marriage & Family Review*, *53*(7), 613–640. https://doi.org/10.1080/01494929.2016.1247761

Polanczyk, G. V., Salum, G. A., Sugaya, L. S., Caye, A., & Rohde, L. A. (2015). Annual research review: A meta-analysis of the worldwide prevalence of mental disorders in children and adolescents. *Journal of Child Psychology and Psychiatry, and Allied Disciplines*, *56*(3), 345–365. https://doi.org/10.1111/jcpp.12381

Racine, N., McArthur, B. A., Cooke, J. E., Eirich, R., Zhu, J., & Madigan, S. (2021). Global prevalence of depressive and anxiety symptoms in children and adolescents during COVID-19: A meta-analysis. *JAMA Pediatrics*, *175*(11), 1142–1150. https://doi.org/10.1001/jamapediatrics.2021.2482

Radez, J., Reardon, T., Creswell, C., Lawrence, P. J., Evdoka-Burton, G., & Waite, P. (2021). Why do children and adolescents (not) seek and access professional help for their mental health problems? A systematic review of quantitative and qualitative studies. *European Child & Adolescent Psychiatry*, *30*(2), 183–211. https://doi.org/10.1007/s00787-019-01469-4

Robinson, L. R., Holbrook, J. R., Bitsko, R. H., Hartwig, S. A., Kaminski, J. W., Ghandour, R., & … Boyle, M. (2017). Differences in health care, family, and community factors associated with mental, behavioral, and developmental disorders among children aged 2–8 years in rural and urban areas, United States, 2011–2012. *MMWR Surveillance Summaries*, *66*(8), 1–11. https://doi.org/10.15585/mmwr.ss6608a1

Rosenzweig, J. M., Barnett, R. C., Huffstutter, K. J., & Stewart, L. M. (2008). Work-life integration: History, theory, and strategy. In J. Rosenzweig & E. Brennan (Eds.), *Work, life, and the mental health system of care: A guide for professionals supporting families of children with emotional or behavioral disorders* (pp. 89–115). Baltimore, MD: Paul H. Brookes.

Roundtree, L., & Lynch, K. (2006). *Exploring the complexities of exceptional caregiving*. Executive briefing series. Boston College, Center for Work & Family.

Samji, H., Wu, J., Ladak, A., Vossen, C., Stewart, E., Dove, N., Long, D., & Snell, G. (2022). Review: Mental health impacts of the COVID-19 pandemic on children and youth – A systematic review. *Child and Adolescent Mental Health*, *27*(2), 173–189. https://doi.org/10.1111/camh.12501

Sellmaier, C., Stewart, L. M., & Brennan, E. M. (2020). Workforce engagement of children and youth with mental health disabilities: The impact of community services and supports. *Community, Work and Family*, *23*(5), 534–555. https://doi.org/10.1080/13668803.2020.1820954

Seltzer, M. M., Greenberg, J. S., Floyd, F. J., Pettee, Y., & Hong, J. (2001). Life course impacts of parenting a child with a disability. *American Journal on Mental Retardation*, *106*(3), 265–286. https://doi.org/10.1352/0895-8017(2001)106<0265:LCIOPA>2.0.CO;2

Splett, J. W. et al (2019). Teacher recognition, concern, and referral of children's internalizing and externalizing behavior problems. *School Mental Health*, *11*(2), 228–239. https://doi.org/10.1007/s12310-018-09303-z.

Stewart, L. M., Sellmaier, C., Brannan, A. M., & Brennan, E. M. (2022). Supporting sleep and health of employed parents with typical and exceptional care demands. *Journal of Social Service Research*, 1–14. https://doi.org/10.1080/01488376.2021.2024935

Stewart, L. M., Sellmaier, C., Brannan, A. M., & Brennan, E. M. (2023). Family demands and workplace supports of employed parents of children with typical and exceptional care responsibilities and their effects on conflict and stress. *Journal of Child and Family Studies*, *32*(4), 1048–1064. https://doi.org/10.1007/s10826-022-02363-5

Teasley, M., McCarter, S., Woo, B., Conner, L. R., Spencer, M. S., & Green, T. (2022). Eliminating racism. In R. P. Barth, J. T. Messing, T. R. Shanks, & J. H. Williams (Eds.), *Grand challenges for social work and society*. Oxford University Press. https://doi.org/10.1093/oso/9780197608043.003.0027

Teicher, M., Samson, J., Anderson, C., & Ohashi, K. (2016). The effects of childhood maltreatment on brain structure, function and connectivity. *Nature Review Neuroscience*, *17*, 652–666. https://doi.org/10.1038/nrn.2016.111

Theule, J., Wiener, J., Tannock, R., & Jenkins, J. M. (2013). Parenting stress in families of children with ADHD: A meta-analysis. *Journal of Child and Family Studies*, *22*(4), 628–642. https://doi.org/10.1177/1063426610387433

Thyberg, C. T., & Lombardi, B. M. (2022). Examining racial differences in internalizing and externalizing diagnoses for children exposed to adverse childhood experiences. *Clinical Social Work Journal, 50*, 286–296. https://doi.org/10.1007/s10615-022-00842-2

U.S. Department of Health and Human Services, Office of the Surgeon General. (2021). *Protecting youth mental health: The U.S. Surgeon General's advisory.* https://www.hhs.gov/sites/default/files/surgeon-general-youth-mental-health-advisory.pdf

Validova, A., Strane, D., Matone, M., Wang, X., Rosenquist, R., Luan, X., & Rubin, D. (2023). Underinsurance among children with special health care needs in the United States. *JAMA Network Open, 6*(12), e2348890. https://doi.org/10.1001/jamanetworkopen.2023.48890

van Eldik, W. M., de Haan, A. D., Parry, L. Q., Davies, P. T., Luijk, M. P. C. M., Arends, L. R., & Prinzie, P. (2020). The interparental relationship: Meta-analytic associations with children's maladjustment and responses to interparental conflict. *Psychological Bulletin, 146*(7), 553–594. https://doi.org/10.1037/bul0000233

Wakefield, J. C., & Conrad, J. A. (2020). Harm as a necessary component of the concept of medical disorder: Reply to Muckler and Taylor. *Journal of Medicine and Philosophy: A Forum for Bioethics and Philosophy of Medicine, 45*(3), 350–370. https://doi.org/10.1093/jmp/jhaa008

Whitney, D. G., & Peterson, M. D. (2019). U.S. National and state-level prevalence of mental health disorders and disparities of mental health care use in children. *JAMA Pediatrics, 173*(4), 389–391. https://doi.org/10.1001/jamapediatrics.2018.5399

Witt, W. P., Gottlieb, C. A., Hampton, J., & Litzelman, K. (2009). The impact of childhood activity limitations on parental health, mental health, and workdays lost. *Academic Pediatrics, 9*(4), 263–269. https://doi.org/10.1016/j.acap.2009.02.008

Wolicki, S. B., Bitsko, R. H., Cree, R. A., Danielson, M. L., Ko, J. Y., Warner, L., & Robinson, L. R. (2021). Mental health of parents and primary caregivers by sex and associated child health indicators. *Adversity and Resilience Science, 2*(2), 125–139. https://doi.org/10.1007/s42844-021-00037-7

World Health Organization (2014). *Social determinants of mental health.* https://www.who.int/publications/i/item/9789241506809

World Health Organization (2019). *ICD-11 for mortality and morbidity statistics (ICD-11 MMS).* https://icd.who.int/en

World Health Organization (2022). *World mental health report: Transforming mental health for all.* World Health Organization. https://www.who.int/publications/i/item/9789240049338

World Health Organization (2023a). *Global health estimates.* https://www.who.int/data/gho/data/themes/mortality-and-global-health-estimates

Zablotsky, B., Ng, A. E., Black, L. I., & Blumberg, S. J. (2023). Diagnosed developmental disabilities in children aged 3-17 years: United States, 2019–2021. *NCHS Data Brief,* (473), 1–8.

2

EXCEPTIONAL CARE AS A SOCIAL JUSTICE ISSUE

Value: *Social Justice*

Ethical Principle: *Social workers challenge social injustice.*

Social workers pursue social change, particularly with and on behalf of vulnerable and oppressed individuals and groups of people. Social workers' social change efforts are focused primarily on issues of poverty, unemployment, discrimination, and other forms of social injustice. These activities seek to promote sensitivity to and knowledge about oppression and cultural and ethnic diversity. Social workers strive to ensure access to needed information, services, and resources; equality of opportunity; and meaningful participation in decision making for all people.

National Association of Social Workers, Code of Ethics (2021)

Social workers commit themselves to a practice of challenging social injustices and furthering social justice. In this chapter, we argue that the barriers parents and families of children with a mental health disability face in their workplaces and communities constitute a social injustice, which must be understood and addressed by social work practitioners, educators, and researchers. As we will discuss in further detail in the following chapters, families face dual stigmatization in the workplace due to the stigmatized nature of mental illness itself, which situates the child's mental health disability as the consequence of bad parenting, and due to the flexibility stigma describing them as bad employees for using workplace flexibilities (Stewart et al., 2024). Employed parents face a greater risk of losing their jobs, having to reduce work hours, or having to forgo promotions, because they lack the support in the workplace or in the community to meet both work and care demands (Sellmaier et al., 2020a). They are therefore at a greater risk for unemployment and poverty. As we learned from parents we interviewed, receiving a diagnosis is not

DOI: 10.4324/9781003532668-2

always accompanied with access to information about treatment options or about how to deal with this news as a couple and family or how and if to disclose any or all of this in the workplace. Parents reported that they have to establish their own support network of peers to learn about their options and rights and have to invest a substantial amount of time and energy into educating themselves (Sellmaier & Buckingham, 2022). In addition, services might not be readily offered or accessed because of health insurance red tape, a lack of providers and long waiting lists, or the inability to take time off during the workday to drive children to appointments. Accessing resources therefore is accompanied by ongoing advocacy. For example, successfully establishing an individual education program does not automatically translate into adequate in-classroom support. All these issues and concerns directly relate to Social Work's Code of Ethics, which states that social change efforts should address poverty, discrimination, and barriers to information and resources.

In this chapter, we will approach exceptional care from a theoretical lens, investigating exceptional care as a social justice issue from three different angles. First, we will take a closer look at different theories related to disability, starting with the medical model of disability. This theoretical approach to understanding disability focuses on the impairment as disabling and uses a deficit lens. The goal of interventions is to fix the individual and help them overcome the limitations imposed by a disability. Next, we will discuss the social model of disability, which was developed by disabled scholars and activists in response to the medical model. This approach situates disability in the social context. The impairment is not considered disabling per se, but the barriers experienced in the social and physical environment when having an impairment are considered disabling. The focus therefore shifts from the individual as lacking to an environment that does not accommodate and is not inclusive. Finally, we will introduce concepts of disability rights, disability justice, and ableism, which further center access as a justice issue. These different theoretical approaches also reflect developments over time with the disability justice movement being the most recent approach to understanding disability, but this does not mean that the medical model is not being used anymore. Depending on the context, one can find all these iterations in workplaces, families, and community systems. We also want to stress that this is not an exhaustive list of disability theories (Hiranandani, 2019) and that the thinking keeps changing with new theories evolving, adding to the complexity of current and future disability theories. We chose to include these theories since they reflect the experiences parents shared with us in our research and because we think that the social model and disability justice approaches can add important impulses for social work practice and social policy development.

Second, we would like to briefly discuss approaching this topic from a rights and from a justice perspective. There is important legislation nationally in the United States and internationally that prohibits discrimination against individuals with disabilities and anyone who is associated with disabled people, such as family members and that enshrines individual's right to employment, education, and community integration. For example, the United Nations Convention on the Rights of Persons with Disabilities was ratified and/or signed by all but six countries (United Nations, n.d.). The Convention explicitly mentions families and family members stating "…that persons with disabilities and their family members should receive the necessary protection and assistance to enable families to contribute toward the full and equal enjoyment of the rights of persons with disabilities" (United Nations, 2006).

BOX 2.1 UNITED NATIONS CONVENTION ON THE RIGHTS OF PERSONS WITH DISABILITIES

In Article 1 of the Convention, mental impairments are explicitly mentioned as a disability included in the Convention. The Convention also explains that full inclusion and participation might be hindered due to societal barriers, making a distinction between the impairment itself and disabling environmental or societal conditions. The United States signed the Convention but has not ratified it yet.

In the following chapters, we will take a deeper look at different policies that can protect families from discrimination and increase access to certain resources. Although legal rights and policies are important tools, they are also at times limited in their reach when trying to address the complexity of exceptional care responsibilities.

Third, as social work researchers, we examine exceptional care from a social work perspective. In addition to the above-discussed connection to the National Association of Social Worker's (NASW) Code of Ethics, we will also introduce social work's Grand Challenges. The Grand Challenges were developed in 2013 under the leadership of the American Academy of Social Work & Social Welfare (AASWSW) and with input from social work scientists, educators, policy experts, and social work organizations. This book specifically ties into and expands on the Grand Challenge of reducing economic insecurity and achieving equal opportunities and justice.

Part 1: Disability Theories

Why disability? When talking about this book, I was asked why we would use disability language when talking about mental health conditions. We think it is therefore critical to share our rationale for talking about mental health disabilities. First, we want to acknowledge that disability especially when viewed from a medical model approach juxtaposes mental health and mental illness or ability and disability with disability being situated outside the norm, a deficit to be ameliorated. If we associate disability with an individual flaw or a shortcoming, then it is understandable to refrain from using the terminology. Movements such as the Hearing Voices movement or terminology such as neurodiversity reflect a distancing from this deficit or disease model. Hearing voices or neurodiversity are considered part of human diversity and not a condition that has to be fixed. At the same time, there are still real-world barriers in education, employment, and community integration. Some consumers or survivors of the psychiatric system experienced human rights violations in the name of helping or curing them, adding an additional layer of complexity to using the disability label. At the same time, some intentionally choose the disability label to reclaim the terminology and to also speak to community and belonging.

BOX 2.2 MORE INFORMATION

You can learn more about the Hearing Voices movement by checking out the Intervoice the International Hearing Voices Movement https://www.intervoiceonline.org/#content or the Hearing Voices Network USA https://www.hearingvoicesusa.org/. In this TedTalk, Eleanor Longden tells her story about the voices in her head and her approach to recovery (https://www.ted.com/talks/eleanor_longden_the_voices_in_my_head).

Within this larger context and discourse, we opted for the use of mental health disability to reflect a critical understanding of disability. If we understand that individuals become disabled because of the barriers, they experience in social and physical spaces, then disability becomes a necessary and helpful lens to better understand the lived experience of individuals with a mental health condition. The goal therefore is to highlight the discrimination still being experienced and to consider disability inclusivity as a social justice issue. Framing exceptional care within this larger context of disability justice draws our attention to the stigmatization and discrimination faced by parents and care providers of children with a mental health disability. School systems that are not inclusive of or accessible for students with mental health needs affect the student and the family as a whole. Workplaces that discriminate against employees with exceptional care responsibilities affect the employee and the family as a whole. Given this complexity and the different individual preferences for language use, we would also like to stress that how an individual identifies and what language they prefer always takes precedence. We opted for language that connects with disability theories and discourses and the use of both person-first and identity-first language in this book to center the still existing discrimination as individuals and families interact with workplaces, communities, and the larger society. Others might opt for different languages and identifiers and in alignment with self-determination, we encourage providers and educators to learn and honor individual's preferences.

In this introduction, we already mentioned the medical and the social model of disability, which we would like to examine more closely in the next section. Looking back in time, the beginnings of the medicalization of ability and disability can be traced back to the Enlightenment era (Gilson & DePoy, 2002). The increasing focus on reasoning, observation, and the mapping of the human body shifted explaining disability as a curse or a moral failure to a physical or mental illness. The medical model of disability builds on this foundation and defines disability as a medical condition or problem to be treated. This perspective opened opportunities for intervention development and treatment opportunities for mental health conditions such as medication or talk therapies, which are an important contribution to our understanding of mental well-being and to supporting individuals with a mental health disability. The limitation and critique of the medical model argue that this approach situates disability within the individual and frames mental illness as an individual deficit or flaw that must be fixed. This can lead to self-blame, shame, and stigmatization. For example, parents reported that they blame themselves and their parenting, or they were blamed by medical providers, family members, and co-workers for their child's disability. A framework that paints the individual with a mental health disability as flawed or defective can also have additional negative effects on the individual's sense of self and overall well-being. A strictly medical interpretation of mental health disabilities therefore situates disability as an individual problem and not as a social justice concern.

The social model of disability was developed in response to these limitations of a medical interpretation of disability. Michael Oliver, a disabled British academic and activist, coined the term social model of disability (Oliver, 2013). This model distinguishes between impairment and disability and argues that individuals with impairments are not disabled because of the specific condition but because of barriers experienced in their physical and social environments. Disability is therefore situated in the interaction between individual and environment and aligns with social work's person-in-environment approach to understanding individual's lives and challenges. Using this lens, we can understand disability as a social justice issue and can work on addressing structural and environmental barriers that hinder individual's well-being and thriving. Maté and Daniel Maté's (2022) understanding of mental health or illness as being a bio-psycho-social response adds another aspect more specific to mental health disabilities. Accordingly, mental illness as an impairment is not just a biological, genetic, or medical concern but must be understood as a response to environmental or societal stressors. Both impairment and disability then have to be understood within the individual's environmental context. It is important to consider some of the critiques of the social model of disability. For example, exactly this distinction between impairment and disability has been considered problematic by some. For example, deaf individuals, neurodiverse individuals, or individuals hearing voices might not think of themselves as having an impairment and would argue that this distinction between impairment and disability reifies the notion or normality with certain human functionings being considered normal and others as impaired. At the same time, others have argued that the social model of disability dismisses the real impact an impairment might have and the challenges and restrictions it might pose independent of the environment.

These two criticisms point to another limitation, which states that disability and the experience of disability are multifaceted and varied. This diversity of experience is not just limited to differences in type of disability but also includes other intersecting identities. For example, a white male identified individual with a mental health disability inhabits different locations of power and oppression than a black female identified individual with a mental health disability. Neither the medical nor the social model of disability includes an explicit analysis of the intersectional experience of privilege and oppression including situating disability as one aspect of an individual's identity among other aspects such as race, ethnicity, gender, sexual orientation, or religious affiliation. Disability justice responds to this critique as a social justice movement centering intersectionality. Patty Berne and Sins Invalid articulated 10 principles of disability justice, including intersectionality, leadership of those most impacted, anti-capitalist politics, cross-movement solidarity, recognizing wholeness, sustainability, commitment to cross-disability solidarity, interdependence, collective access, and collective liberation (Sins Invalid, n.d.).

Part 2: Disability: Rights and Justice

The work of the disability justice movement also broadens the conversation from a rights focus to a broader justice framework. In the United States during the 1960s and 1970s people with different disabilities organized to fight for the removal of barriers to societal participation and for the rights for full inclusion in education, employment, housing, and other societal institutions (American Association of People with Disabilities, n.d.). Organizing for political change aligns with the theoretical framework of the social model introduced above. The understanding that disability is situated in systems and societal structures calls for solutions that bring about political and social change. The disability rights movement in the United States was instrumental for passing the Americans with Disabilities Act (ADA) in 1990.

BOX 2.3 ADA DEFINITION OF DISABILITY

In Chapter 126, Section 12102 of the Americans with Disabilities Act, disability is defined as:

A *a physical or mental impairment that substantially limits one or more major life activities of such individual;*
B *a record of such an impairment; or*
C *being regarded as having such an impairment*

Section 12112 also explicitly protects individuals who are associated with an individual with a disability from employment-based discrimination.

We will talk more about the ADA and how it relates to exceptional care in Chapter 6. The disability justice movement adds to this political work and perspective arguing that a rights-focused approach is too narrow. Rights as state-sanctioned responses to discrimination are important but not sufficient to create just spaces and societies. For example, the right to accommodations in higher education can create conditions for students with a mental health condition to attend and graduate from college, but accessing accommodations can be difficult (Sellmaier & Kim, 2021). For example, students need a medical diagnosis to access accommodations, which requires health insurance, and some required testing might not be covered by health insurance. Accommodations are also often not individualized and can be limited in their benefit. For example, extra time on tests or assignment extensions might not be sufficient if a student is in a mental health crisis. Accommodations are also difficult to translate into a practicum setting when considering social work education specifically. In its current version, it is also incumbent on the disabled individual not only to ask for the accommodations but also to sue organizations and institutions if they violate the rights guaranteed by the ADA, a process that is time intensive, stressful, and requires financial resources. The focus therefore is to adjust systems and institutions to enable access as far as is "reasonable," but a rights-approach does not necessarily question the structures and expectations at the root of these institutions.

BOX 2.4 DEFINITION

Some distinguish between ableism as discrimination in favor of non-disabled individuals and disableism as discrimination against disabled individuals (Scope https://www.scope.org.uk/about-us/disablism). And sometimes ableism is broadly defined as discrimination against individuals due to their disability (Smith, Center for Disability Rights https://cdrnys.org/blog/uncategorized/ableism/). This discrimination includes individual behaviors and beliefs, and institutional barriers, such as assuming a disabled individual is less capable, not hiring them because of their disability, or buildings without ramps or elevators.

The disability justice movement on the other hand identifies anti-capitalist politics as one of its core principles, questioning notions of constant productivity, for example. Our value in a capitalist society is tied to our productive output usually in the form of full-time employment. Anyone not meeting these expectations can be stigmatized as lazy and not deserving. A just and anti-ableist society therefore assures that individuals have access to meaningful work no matter their abilities and that meaningful contributions are multifaceted going beyond capitalist understandings of work and productivity. A justice-focused approach also brings solutions into view that are not limited to legal rights and government responses, such as mutual aid. Individuals rely on friends and family-members to provide care for example, especially in a society with limited community-based services and resources.

Disabled individuals also support each other and care for each other, care work that often goes unacknowledged in a society that frames disabled individuals often as helpless and needy (Piepzna-Samarasinha & Wong, 2019).

We would like to reiterate that this discussion of different disability theories and approaches to disability advocacy is not exhaustive but only provides an overview. The end of this chapter provides a list of resources and additional material for a deeper exploration.

Part 3: Exceptional Care in the Context of Disability Theories

Our book focuses on parents and families of children with a mental health disability and their access to workplace and community resources. The question therefore is how do these theories and approaches connect to the topic of exceptional care.

BOX 2.5 DEFINITION OF EXCEPTIONAL CARE

Exceptional care responsibilities are any type of care responsibilities that go beyond typical care responsibilities. This can include caring for aging parents while caring for children, caring for an ill spouse, or caring for a child with a disability. Exceptional care responsibilities are often crisis-driven, require substantial time managing services and care, and continue beyond childhood and adolescence (Roundtree & Lynch, 2006). As mentioned in Chapter 1, these care responsibilities can impact families' economic and work situation, their social relationships, and their physical and mental health.

First, a social model lens identifies the barriers and struggles families face as situated within the environment. Exceptional care responsibilities can be challenging in and of itself, but they are being exacerbated by certain structural and environmental conditions. For example, as a parent, I worry about my child's ability to keep up with schoolwork, to develop healthy relationships, or my child being bullied in school. Some of these worries might be triggered or increased in an ableist society, when parents only hear messaging about the importance of perfect grades in a race to get into the best college, in a society with a limited social safety net and a job market that often requires a college degree to make a living wage. In addition to the emotional toll, the lack of workplace flexibility, paid time off to manage health crises, waiting lists to get an appointment with a mental health professional, or schools that don't have the training or resources to effectively address behavioral concerns, can create instrumental barriers that make parenting with exceptional care responsibilities so much more challenging, time consuming, and stressful.

Second, the discussion of rights and justice applies to exceptional care as well. Rights such as protection from discrimination based on family care responsibilities, access to Family Medical Leave, or the right to free and quality public education for all children are critical and need further expansion. At the same time, families already use mutual aid and support each other with practical tips, child care, and emotional support, all mechanisms that go beyond institutional and political solutions. In addition, supporting families to thrive requires an examination of our underlying societal assumptions of the role of the family, of the value of care work especially in contrast to paid work. These questions ask us how we envision a just society that enables access, equitable opportunities, and meaningful participation for all. The following chapters examine more closely families' experience in workplace, family, and community systems, discussing legal frameworks that create certain rights for families and individuals as well as the role of mutual care. Furthermore, the descriptions of the role of workplaces and communities will underscore a social model of disability centering on how a family's context and environment affects their exceptional care experience.

Part 4: Social Work Ethics and the Grand Challenges

As social workers, the NASW Code of Ethics (2021) or the ethical principles of the International Federation of Social Workers (2018) serve as guidelines for analyzing and envisioning just and equitable conditions. Both of these frameworks stipulate that the primary mission of social work is to improve the lives of individuals and of society as a whole, specifically mentioning that individual well-being is considered within the social context. The values of social justice, self-determination, participation, and dignity are central to social work. These values are also clearly relevant for working with parents with exceptional care responsibilities. Exceptional care responsibilities and more specifically the lack of support can increase the risk for unemployment or underemployment, limiting self-determination and participation of family members (Sellmaier et al., 2020b). Parents and individuals with mental health disabilities experience stigmatization and discrimination, which often results in exclusion and negatively affects well-being (Sellmaier & Buckingham, 2022). Respecting the dignity of every person asks social workers to support self-determination, human dignity, and equal access to opportunities. This is predicated on having opportunities to choose from, which requires that we ensure access to resources that allow families to thrive at home, at work, and in their communities.

BOX 2.6 THE GRAND CHALLENGES FOR SOCIAL WORK

The Grand Challenges for Social Work were first developed in 2013 by a committee consisting of social work scientists, educators, and policy experts. The committee sought input from social work organizations and academic groups. The original 80 concepts were summarized and synthesized to 12 Grand Challenges. The Grand Challenges are separated in three broad categories including individual and family well-being, stronger social fabric, and just society. Each of these broader categories includes several subthemes.

TABLE 2.1 Grand Challenges

Individual and family well-being	*Stronger social fabric*	*Just society*
Ensure healthy development for youth	Eradicate social isolation	Eliminate racism
Close the health gap	End homelessness	Promote smart decarceration
Build healthy relationships to end violence	Create social responses to a changing environment	Build financial capability and assets for all
Advance long and productive lives	Harness technology for social good	Reduce extreme economic inequality
	Prevent gun violence	Achieve equal opportunity and justice

Social work's Grand Challenges (2026) spearheaded by the AASWSW provide some helpful details to the understanding and political implications of current social problems. We would like to highlight *reducing economic inequality* and *achieving equal opportunity and justice* for their relevance to issues of exceptional care. Economic inequality has been growing in the United States over the last decades with hourly wages for the lowest incomes declining and for most other households' wages stagnating or changing only minimally (Lein et al., 2016). In contrast, income produced by capital has increased while income produced by labor has not increased or even decreased. This is also accompanied by a widening gap in the quality of jobs with good jobs offering stability, flexible schedules, and benefits such as health insurance and paid time off. Low-income households do not just face lower-paying jobs, but also often cannot rely on stable schedules but face on-demand hourly hiring practices with limited options for reliable and family-driven flexibility, and with no or limited access to benefits such as paid leave or retirement benefits. Exceptional care responsibilities are an additional compounding factor when considering economic inequality. Parents are more likely to have to reduce work hours, forgo promotions, or give up work altogether, since their workplace demands cannot be integrated with their care demands (Sellmaier et al., 2020b). Jobs without benefits such as health care or paid time off pose additional challenges, since access to adequate medical treatment is critical, and the likelihood for the need to take time off to deal with a medical crisis is increased. Reduced income and the increased costs for out-of-pocket payments, treatments, or equipment raise the risk for impoverishment (Blackwell, 2025; Lynch & Dickerson, 2012). The cost and availability of child care in the United States is another factor playing into economic inequality. As we will discuss in Chapter 6, finding and maintaining affordable and quality child care is even more difficult for families of children with mental health needs, and depending on the nature of the disability additional after-school care beyond the elementary and middle school years might be required. Economic insecurity increases the challenges to meet exceptional care responsibilities. At the same time, exceptional care responsibilities increase the risk for economic insecurity. Addressing this Grand Challenge of economic inequality therefore clearly aligns with a call for a deeper understanding and for better support of families with exceptional care responsibilities.

The Grand Challenge of achieving equal opportunity and justice is also highly relevant to issues of exceptional care. The authors for this Grand Challenge identify historic and present-day discrimination and stigmatization as barriers to equal opportunities for all, including access to employment (Goldbach et al., 2015). Social work research is called to examine the factors that contribute to inequity and exclusion and to develop policies and programs to fight discrimination and to increase equal access to education, health care, housing, and employment. The work on reducing discrimination by addressing social stigma is especially relevant for this book. As we will discuss in greater detail in later chapters, parents of children with mental health disabilities experience courtesy stigma or stigma by association (Stewart et al., 2024). Stereotypes about mental health conditions can be especially insidious since parents are often blamed for their child's condition or blame themselves. Parents can also experience flexibility stigma, since they might be pegged as unreliable workers. This is especially prevalent for fathers taking family-related leaves or other workplace flexibilities due to care work, since these fathers neither conform with ideal worker norms nor with gendered expectations for care work. Considering courtesy and flexibility stigma and the discrimination associated with it offers therefore an important addition or expansion of social work's call to dismantling social stigmatization.

Part 5: Summary: Exceptional Care as a Social Justice Issue

In summary, exceptional care responsibilities can be conceptualized as a social justice issue, which aligns with social work's mission. Critical disability theories such as the social model of disability and the disability justice movement provide an important lens to understanding both disability and exceptional care. Parents caring for a child with a mental health disability experience social and structural barriers in their workplaces and their communities. Situating exceptional care as a social justice issue draws attention to these structural barriers and advocates for changes that go beyond individual rehabilitation or adjustment. Exceptional care is not the problem, but families struggle because they are not well supported. In addition, rights can only be one part of the solution if we think of exceptional care as a social justice issue. They are a very important aspect of the solution, but as pointed out by the disability justice movement, they also fall short. For example, parents are protected against discrimination by the Americans with Disabilities Act, but this legislation alone does not stop stigmatizing and discriminatory behavior and actions in the workplace. Situating exceptional care within a justice framework therefore provides a specific lens for examining employment, work-life fit, and access to community resources for these families, a lens that focuses on societal and structural barriers. It also allows us to pay attention to sites of struggle and resistance, of peer support and mutual aid to remove barriers and to thrive.

- Families with exceptional care responsibilities experience discrimination and barriers to full participation in work and society, making exceptional care responsibilities a social justice issue.
- The social model of disability clarifies that individuals with a mental health condition are disabled because of environmental barriers and stigmatization that hinder full participation.
- Rights for equitable treatment and protection from discrimination are critical, and a justice focus broadens our lens to examine access to resources and approaches to mutual aid beyond limiting ourselves to governmental responses alone.

Part 6: Implications for Social Work Practice

The connections with the social work ethical codes and the Grand Challenges of social work demonstrate that exceptional care responsibilities are part of social work's mission and should be considered when working with individuals and when engaging in organizational and policy change efforts. For example, considering barriers to services or why parents might not show up to meetings is important for any agency or organization that works with children. In conversations with school personnel, I often heard that parents don't care about their child's education because they don't show up for meetings. I also heard from parents that IEP meetings or other school consultations often took place during parents' work hours, and attending them can put them at risk for losing their job or for reprimands from their supervisors. Similarly, a social work practitioner who provides mental health services to a child should understand the intersection of work and care demands for parents to better serve the child and the family as a whole. Parents might struggle with dropping their child off for appointments in time, because they work and can't easily leave their workplace during work hours. This behavior can easily be interpreted as parents being disengaged or not caring about their child's health, if we are unaware of the multiple demands parents face. An understanding of disability theories and of exceptional care responsibilities can be a helpful lens to examine our services for access barriers and to improve accessibility. In later chapters, we will discuss the more practical impacts of exceptional care responsibilities on families and how workplaces and community services can support families, but disability theories can be an important tool to understand and ameliorate social work service access issues. Adding exceptional care as a social and disability justice issue to the social work curriculum will ensure a workforce that is educated about and competent to effectively work with families who care for a child with a mental health disability. Our curriculum right now often only provides limited content on disability issues (Ogden et al., 2017) especially when we consider a more critical understanding of disability issues and theories (Kim & Sellmaier, 2019).

- Critical disability theories provide a more holistic understanding for social work practitioners.
- Critical disability theories move practitioners away from deficit-oriented models aligning practice with a strength perspective.
- Disability-related content has to be strengthened in social work education to prepare practitioners for anti-ableist practice.

Part 7: Application for Social Work Education

Understanding exceptional care as a social justice issue bears several important implications for social work education. In general, exceptional care responsibilities should be included in course work that is focused on Council on Social Work Educations (CSWE) 2022 Educational Policy and Assessment Standards Competency 2 *Advance Human Rights and Social, Racial, Economic, and Environmental Justice* and Competency 3 *Engage Anti-Racism, Diversity, Equity, and Inclusion (ADEI) in Practice.* Instructors can include a discussion of exceptional care responsibilities in their courses to identify how exceptional care responsibilities or the discrimination associated with these care situations result in economic and social injustice. This is a critical first step, since disability content and a critical analysis of disability and its associated care is often still absent from social work education. The following activities offer some concrete examples on working with this chapter's content in different types of classes.

ACTIVITY: APPLYING DISABILITY THEORIES TO A CASE SCENARIO

Competency 6: Engage with Individuals, Families, Groups, Organizations, and Communities

Competency 7: Assess Individuals, Families, Groups, Organizations, and Communities

Competency 8: Intervene with Individuals, Families, Groups, Organizations, and Communities

TABLE 2.2 Activity—Applying Disability Theories to a Case Scenario

Medical model	*Social model*
Focus on the individual	Focus on individual within social environment
Disability is considered a within-individual condition	Disability is considered an in-between individual and environment condition
Focus on diagnosis, treatment, and prevention	Assess and ameliorate environmental conditions to increase access and inclusion

Case scenario:

You are a school social worker in a middle school, and you work with 13-year-old Toby. Toby has been struggling in his classes. He has a hard time sitting still and focusing on the teacher. He stands up frequently, and he does not follow the teacher's instructions. He often misses his homework and his notebook for class. He is socially isolated and seems to have few friends in class. He can get angry at times with his classmates, which makes it harder to connect with them. The teacher frequently sends Toby to your office, when he disrupts the classroom. He has missed much of the class work, because of that. The teacher has tried to meet with Toby's parents, but it is difficult to find a time that works for them or they cancel meetings short-notice. You know from Toby that both his parents work full-time. They are self-employed and run a small corner store. They don't have any employees and have to manage everything themselves. Toby also has three younger siblings.

Questions:

- If you use a medical model approach to understand Toby's situation, what information would you focus on?
- If you use a social model approach, what information would you focus on then?
- What similarities and differences do you notice in your understanding of Toby's situation based on the two approaches?
- What are the benefits and limitations of each approach?
- What would be your intervention plan if you consider only information from one approach, and what would be your intervention plan if you consider information from both the medical and the social model?

ACTIVITY: UNDERSTANDING DISABILITY RIGHTS

Competency 2: Advance Human Rights and Social, Racial, Economic, and Environmental Justice
Competency 3: Engage Anti-Racism, Diversity, Equity, and Inclusion (ADEI) in Practice
Competency 5: Engage in Policy Practice

Learn more about the disability rights movement by watching the documentary *Lives worth Living* (2011). Discuss the following questions:

- What does the documentary teach you about disability history, theory, and how the different systems such as housing, education, or employment are impacted by disability?
- How does the social model of disability help you understand the struggles described in the documentary?
- What were the problems triggering the disability rights movement?
- What did activists do to initiate change?

ACTIVITY: UNDERSTANDING THE SOCIAL WORK CONTEXT

Competency 2: Advance Human Rights and Social, Racial, Economic, and Environmental Justice
Competency 5: Engage in Policy Practice
Competency 8: Intervene with Individuals, Families, Groups, Organizations, and Communities

Explore the Grand Challenges for Social Work and select one of the grand challenges.

- Read the concept paper to learn more about this specific grand challenge.
- Summarize the main arguments of the concept paper, including the policy and intervention recommendations.
- What connections can you make between the Grand Challenge you selected and the issues discussed in this chapter?

Resource List

Disability Visibility Project: https://disabilityvisibilityproject.com/
Documentary about the Disability Justice Movement called *Lives Worth Living* (2011). https://www.pbs.org/independentlens/documentaries/lives-worth-living/
Grand Challenges for Social Work: https://grandchallengesforsocialwork.org/
International Federation of Social Workers: Global Social Work Statement of Ethical Principles: https://www.ifsw.org/global-social-work-statement-of-ethical-principles/
National Association of Social Workers: Code of Ethics: https://www.socialworkers.org/About/Ethics/Code-of-Ethics/Code-of-Ethics-English
Sins Invalid: https://sinsinvalid.org/
United Nations' Convention on the Rights of Persons with Disabilities: https://www.ohchr.org/en/instruments-mechanisms/instruments/convention-rights-persons-disabilities

References

American Association of People with Disabilities (n.d.). The movement for disability rights and justice. Retrieved from: https://www.aapd.com/movement/

Blackwell, C. (2025). The impact of school challenges on parental employment among families with children on the autism spectrum. *Disability & Society*, *40*(2), 235–253. https://doi.org/10.1080/09687599.2024.2313096

Gilson, S. F., & DePoy, E. (2002). Theoretical approaches to disability content in social work education. *Journal of Social Work Education*, *38*(1), 153–165. https://doi.org/10.1080/10437797.2002.10779088

Goldbach, J. T., Amaro, H., Vega, W., & Walter, M. D. (2015). The Grand Challenge of promoting equality by addressing social stigma. *Grand Challenges for Social Work Initiative.* Retrieved from: https://grandchallengesforsocialwork.org/wp-content/uploads/2016/01/W16-The-Grand-Challenge-of-Promoting-Equality-by-Addressing-Social-Stigma1-1-2.pdf

Hiranandani, V. (2019). Towards a critical theory of disability in social work. *Critical Social Work, 6*(1). https://doi.org/10.22329/csw.v6i1.5712
International Federation of Social Workers (2018). Global social work statement of ethical principles. Retrieved from: https://www.ifsw.org/global-social-work-statement-of-ethical-principles/
Kim, J., & Sellmaier, C. (2019). Making disability visible in social work education. *Journal of Social Work Education, 56*(3), 496–507. https://doi.org/10.1080/10437797.2019.1661899
Lein, L., Romich, J. L., & Sherraden, M. (2016). Reversing extreme inequality. *Grand Challenges for Social Work Initiative*. Retrieved from: https://grandchallengesforsocialwork.org/wp-content/uploads/2016/01/WP16-with-cover-2.pdf
Lynch, F., & Dickerson, J. (2012). PS2-21: Validity and reliability of the family economic impact interview: A new instrument to measure costs related to child mental health conditions. *Clinical Medical Research, 10*(3), 1–81.
Maté, G., & Maté, D. (2022). *The myth of normal : Trauma, illness, & healing in a toxic culture*. Avery, an imprint of Penguin Random House.
National Association of Social Workers. (2021). Code of ethics. Retrieved from: https://www.socialworkers.org/About/Ethics/Code-of-Ethics/Code-of-Ethics-English
Ogden, L., McAllister, C., & Neely-Barnes, S. (2017). Assessment of integration of disability content into social work education. *Journal of Social Work in Disability & Rehabilitation, 16*(3–4), 361–376. https://doi.org/10.1080/1536710X.2017.1392394
Oliver, M. (2013). The social model of disability. Thirty years on. *Disability and Society, 28*(7), 1024–1026. https://doi.org/10.1080/09687599.2013.818773
Piepzna-Samarasinha, L. L., & Wong, A. (2019). Disability Visibility Podcast: Episode 48: Care Work. Retrieved from: https://disabilityvisibilityproject.com/2019/04/07/ep-48-care-work/
Roundtree, L., & Lynch, K. (2006). *Exploring the complexities of exceptional caregiving. Executive briefing series*. Boston College, Center for Work & Family.
Sellmaier, C., & Buckingham, S. (2022). "I think sometimes that dads are kind of forgotten (…) so it's nice that we also get a voice.": Work-life experiences of employed U.S. fathers caring for a child with special health care needs. *Community, Work, & Family, 25*(5), 661–676. https://doi.org/10.1080/13668803.2021.1911935
Sellmaier, C., & Kim, J. (2021). Disability accommodation experiences of social work students in the United States. *Social Work Education: The International Journal, 40*(7), 872–887. https://doi.org/10.1080/02615479.2020.1738375
Sellmaier, C., Stewart, L., Brennan, E. M., Rosenzweig, J. M, & Malsch, A. M. (2020a). Disabilities and work-family challenges: Parents having children with special healthcare needs. *Work Family Researchers Network Encyclopedia.* https://wfrn.org/encyclopedia/parents-of-children-and-youth-with-disabilities-providing-exceptional-care-and-meeting-work-life-challenges/
Sellmaier, C., Stewart, L. M., & Brennan, E. M. (2020b). Workforce engagement of parents of children and youth with mental health difficulties: The impact of community services and supports. *Community Work & Family, 23*(5), 534–555. https://doi.org/10.1080/13668803.2020.1820954
Sins Invalid (n.d.). 10 principles of disability justice. Retrieved from: https://sinsinvalid.org/10-principles-of-disability-justice/
Stewart, L., Sellmaier, C., Henderson-Posther, M., Brennan, E. M., & Lukefahr, J. (2024). Navigating family responsibility discrimination: Parenting a child with a mental health disability. I: P. Neff Claster, & S. L. Blair: *Contemporary perspectives in family research, 27*. Emerald Publishing.
United Nations (n.d.). Status of ratification: Interactive dashboard. Retrieved from: https://indicators.ohchr.org/
United Nations (2006). Convention on the Rights of Persons with Disabilities. Retrieved from: https://www.ohchr.org/en/instruments-mechanisms/instruments/convention-rights-persons-disabilities

3

THE COMMUNITY, WORK, AND FAMILY INTERFACE

Theoretical Analysis

Parenting a child with a mental health disability takes place within the interconnected contexts of family life, employment, and community systems. For parents, caregiving is not limited to managing symptoms or accessing treatment. It also involves coordinating school responses, navigating health and social service systems, maintaining employment, and responding to crises that often arise without warning (Brannan et al., 2018). These responsibilities shape parents' daily lives and long-term trajectories, influencing family well-being, economic stability, and health outcomes (Bitsko, 2022; Sellmaier et al., 2020a, 2021).

This chapter argues that parenting a child with a mental health disability cannot be adequately understood through traditional work–family or family systems theories alone (Brown & Clark, 2017; Stewart et al., 2018). Existing frameworks often assume predictable caregiving trajectories, stable role boundaries, and institutional supports that can be planned for and negotiated in advance (Kossek & Thompson, 2016; Moen, 2011; Voydanoff, 2005). In contrast, parenting a child with a mental health disability is frequently characterized by cyclical crises, heightened stigma, and misalignment between caregiving demands and available supports (Roundtree & Lynch, 2006; Sellmaier et al., 2020b).

Social workers across practice settings regularly encounter parents who are struggling to balance these intersecting demands. In schools, healthcare settings, community agencies, and workplaces, social workers support families facing service fragmentation, stigma, and limited institutional flexibility. Parents may miss work due to school exclusions, emergency appointments, or behavioral crises, negotiate whether and how to disclose their child's mental health needs to employers, or reduce or leave employment altogether when available supports fail to align with caregiving demands (Sellmaier et al., 2020b; Stewart & Charles, 2022). These experiences are not individual anomalies. They reflect

DOI: 10.4324/9781003532668-3

broader structural conditions that shape how care, work, and family life intersect (Brannan et al., 2022).

Table 3.1 provides a structured overview of the theoretical frameworks informing this chapter and illustrates how each can be operationalized in social work practice across micro, mezzo, and macro levels.

Part 1: Situating Exceptional Care in Relation to Other Life Roles

Parenting a child with a mental health disability occurs within the interconnected contexts of family life, employment, and community systems (Rosenzweig et al., 2008; Sellmaier et al., 2020a). For parents, caregiving extends far beyond managing symptoms or accessing treatment. It encompasses ongoing coordination with schools, navigation of fragmented health and social service systems, crisis response, and sustained advocacy on behalf of their child (Brennan et al., 2016). These responsibilities unfold alongside expectations associated with employment, partnership, and community participation, shaping parents' daily experiences and long-term trajectories.

Exceptional care also differs from typical care in its complexity (Stewart et al., 2018). Parents must develop specialized knowledge, coordinate among multiple service systems, and engage in continuous decision-making about disclosure, advocacy, and risk (Stewart et al., 2025). These demands are compounded by stigma, which can constrain access to informal supports and make reliance on formal systems contingent on revealing sensitive information about a child's mental health (Rosenzweig et al., 2011; Stewart & Charles, 2022). From a social work perspective, situating care in relation to other life roles requires attending not only to the child's needs but also to the cumulative strain placed on parents as caregivers, workers, and community members. Social workers across school, healthcare, community, and employment settings are often positioned at the intersections of these roles. Understanding exceptional care as a structuring condition of parents' lives, rather than an individual or temporary disruption, is essential for meaningful assessment, intervention, and advocacy (Brannan et al., 2022; Stewart et al., 2025).

Role Theory and the Work–Family Interface

Role theory (Pleck, 1997) provides a foundational framework for understanding how parents experience conflict when competing expectations associated with caregiving and employment collide. Individuals occupy multiple social roles, each governed by norms related to time, behavior, and commitment. Work–family conflict arises when demands from the work role interfere with family responsibilities, while family–work conflict occurs when caregiving demands disrupt employment obligations (Greenhaus & Beutell, 1985). From a work–family fit perspective, these conflicts signal misalignment between role demands and available resources across work, family, and community systems (Voydanoff, 2005). Role theory is

TABLE 3.1 Theory to Practice Integration: Framework's Guiding Social Work with Parents of Children with Mental Health Disabilities

Theoretical framework	*Key constructs and concepts*	*Illustrative research (2010–2025)*	*Social work implications (micro, mezzo, macro)*
Life Course Theory (Elder, 1998)	Trajectories, transitions, turning points, cumulative disadvantage, linked lives	Stewart et al. (2024); Namkung et al. (2015)	**Micro:** Assess caregiving transitions and crisis points that shape cumulative stress and opportunity structures. **Mezzo:** Design anticipatory supports during key family transitions (e.g., diagnosis, school changes, adolescence). **Macro:** Advocate for lifespan-informed service systems and parental leave policies that account for recurring care crises.
Border/Boundary Theory (Ashforth et al., 2000; Clark, 2000)	Boundary permeability, segmentation/integration, border-crossing strategies, role strain	Rosenzweig et al. (2011); Stewart and Charles (2022)	**Micro:** Support clients in developing boundary management skills and safe disclosure strategies at work. **Mezzo:** Educate employers and supervisors about family-supportive organizational practices. **Macro:** Advance policies promoting flexible work arrangements and caregiver protection legislation.
Ecological Systems/ Ecological Fit Theory (Bronfenbrenner, 1979; Voydanoff, 2005)	Micro-meso-macro interactions, demands/ resources balance, proximal processes	Sellmaier (2019b)	**Micro:** Assess the match between family needs and available community supports. **Mezzo:** Build collaborative care networks linking schools, employers, and service providers. **Macro:** Advocate for systemic coordination across health, education, and employment systems to reduce fragmentation.
Family Systems–Illness Model (Rolland, 1993)	Family meaning-making, role reorganization, chronic illness trajectory, family development stage	Sellmaier and Buckingham (2022); Stewart et al. (2025)	**Micro:** Facilitate family meaning-making and adaptive coping strategies around a child's mental health diagnosis. **Mezzo:** Develop group interventions that strengthen family communication and cohesion. **Macro:** Promote family-centered models in mental health and disability policy and funding frameworks.

(*Continued*)

TABLE 3.1 (Continued)

Theoretical framework	*Key constructs and concepts*	*Illustrative research (2010–2025)*	*Social work implications (micro, mezzo, macro)*
Stigma Theory (Goffman, 1963)	Felt/enacted stigma, courtesy stigma, identity management, disclosure, and concealment	Liegghio (2017); Stewart et al. (2025)	**Micro:** Use stigma-informed assessment to validate parent experiences and reduce internalized blame. **Mezzo:** Partner with parent organizations to develop anti-stigma workplace and school initiatives. **Macro:** Address structural stigma through equity legislation and public education campaigns.
Continuum of Dependent Care Model (Stewart et al., 2018)	Typical vs. exceptional care, care intensity, complexity, and typology, resource gains/losses	Stewart et al. (2018, 2022); Sellmaier (2019a)	**Micro:** Assess where a family falls on the care continuum to tailor interventions and supports. **Mezzo:** Design workplace and community interventions that align resources with caregiving intensity. **Macro:** Inform policy development to address caregiver inequities across service and employment systems.
Conservation of Resources Theory (COR) (Hobfoll, 2011; applied in Stewart et al., 2022)	Resource loss/gain cycles, stress buffering, organizational and social resources	Stewart et al. (2022); Stewart et al. (2024)	**Micro:** Build caregiver resilience through resource-focused interventions and skills training. **Mezzo:** Develop organizational cultures that prevent caregiver resource depletion. **Macro:** Use evidence on caregiver resource inequities to support legislative action on paid leave, respite, and flexible work protections.

therefore useful for identifying where strain originates when parents attempt to meet expectations in multiple domains simultaneously.

However, role theory alone is insufficient for explaining the experiences of parents raising children with mental health disabilities. Empirical research demonstrates that exceptional caregiving introduces chronic, unpredictable, and crisis-driven demands that fundamentally alter how role conflict is experienced and sustained over time (Rosenzweig et al., 2011; Sellmaier et al., 2016; Stewart, 2013). Unlike parents managing typical caregiving trajectories, parents of children with mental health disabilities face recurrent disruptions that make role negotiation an ongoing condition rather than an episodic challenge (Rosenzweig et al., 2002). These dynamics reveal a key limitation of traditional role theory: it identifies the presence of conflict but does not account for how stigma, institutional inflexibility, and service fragmentation constrain parents' ability to adapt roles or restore fit. As Brown and Clark (2017) argue, disability-related caregiving requires theoretical frameworks that move beyond role strain to examine how structural conditions shape parents' capacity to remain employed, access supports, and sustain family well-being.

Part 2: Life Course, Boundaries, and Ecological Contexts in Parenting a Child with a Mental Health Disability

Life course theory (Elder, 1998) provides a temporal lens for understanding how parenting a child with a mental health disability unfolds across time and through key transitions. Rather than viewing caregiving as a static role, life course theory emphasizes trajectories, turning points, and cumulative advantage or disadvantage shaped by historical, social, and institutional contexts (Elder, 1998). For parents of children with mental health disabilities, caregiving trajectories are frequently punctuated by unexpected crises, diagnostic milestones, school transitions, service disruptions, and periods of acute instability that require rapid adaptation (Stewart et al., 2018, 2024).

These transitions do not occur in isolation. Parents' lives are characterized by what Elder (1998) referred to as *linked lives*, in which a child's mental health needs are deeply intertwined with parental employment, health, and identity. Disruptions in one domain, such as school exclusion, repeated behavioral crises, or loss of services, can cascade into employment instability, financial strain, and deteriorating health, shaping long-term trajectories of risk or resilience (Brannan et al., 2022; Sellmaier et al., 2020). Over time, these repeated disruptions accumulate, producing cumulative disadvantage when institutional supports are insufficient or inaccessible, particularly for families facing stigma, immigration-related barriers, or socioeconomic precarity (Stewart et al., 2024).

Boundary and border theories complement life course perspectives by focusing on how parents manage the ongoing negotiation between work, family, and community roles in real time (Ashforth et al., 2000; Clark, 2000). Boundaries between domains are socially constructed and vary in their permeability, flexibility, and legitimacy. For parents of children with mental health disabilities, boundaries are often highly permeable due to crisis-driven demands, such as urgent calls from schools, sudden service needs, or behavioral emergencies that require immediate parental response (Rosenzweig et al., 2008). Managing these boundaries involves active and continuous decision-making about disclosure, integration, and segmentation (Rosenzweig et al., 2011). Parents must weigh the benefits of accessing workplace flexibility and support against the risks of stigma, discrimination, or career penalty associated with revealing a child's mental health needs (Rosenzweig et al., 2011; Stewart & Charles, 2022).

Recent research further demonstrates that these disclosure decisions are shaped not only by workplace culture but also by parents' prior experiences of support or retaliation, contributing to increasingly cautious boundary strategies over time. When workplaces lack flexibility or understanding, boundary strain intensifies, increasing stress and limiting parents' capacity to sustain employment (Brannan et al., 2022; Stewart et al., 2022). In work–family integration terms, boundary permeability reflects parents' efforts to integrate caregiving and employment roles in pursuit of fit, while enforced segmentation through concealment or inflexible workplaces often exacerbates misfit rather than resolving it (Ashforth et al., 2000; Stewart & Charles, 2022; Voydanoff, 2005).

Ecological systems theory, and specifically ecological fit perspectives, situate these boundary negotiations within broader institutional contexts (Bronfenbrenner, 1979; Voydanoff, 2005). Parents operate within interconnected systems that include family, workplace, school, healthcare, and policy environments. Well-being is influenced not simply by the presence of supports but by the fit between caregiving demands and available resources across these systems (Kossek et al., 2022). For parents of children with mental health disabilities, access to resources is often contingent on disclosure of their child's mental health status, fragmented eligibility criteria, or inconsistent institutional responses, producing persistent ecological misfit.

Taken together, life course theory explains when caregiving demands intensify and accumulate, boundary and border theories explain how parents negotiate competing role expectations and disclosure decisions in real time, and ecological fit theory explains why stress and inequity emerge when institutional supports fail to align with caregiving realities. For parents of children with mental health disabilities, these processes operate simultaneously rather than sequentially, producing cycles of crisis, adaptation, and resource gain or loss that shape parental health, employment trajectories, and family well-being across time (Stewart et al., 2018).

From a work–family perspective, these disruptions represent moments of fit breakdown, when caregiving demands exceed available resources across work, family, and community systems (Sellmaier, 2019a; Voydanoff, 2005). Parents are not passive recipients of these breakdowns but actively engage in strategies aimed at restoring fit, including renegotiating work schedules, drawing on family flexibility, coordinating services, or altering boundary permeability. For parents of children with mental health disabilities, however, opportunities to restore fit are often constrained by stigma, fragmented eligibility criteria, and inconsistent institutional responses, transforming short-term misalignment into persistent misfit (Brown & Clark, 2017; Kossek et al., 2022; Stewart, 2013).

Part 3: Disability, Stigma, and Family Adaptation in Parenting a Child with a Mental Health Disability

Disability theory provides a critical lens for understanding how parenting a child with a mental health disability is shaped not only by caregiving demands but also by social, cultural, and institutional responses to disability itself (Corrigan & Miller, 2004). Within social work, disability frameworks challenge medicalized and individualizing interpretations of distress and instead emphasize how stigma, discrimination, and structural barriers constrain family well-being, participation, and access to resources across social domains. For parents of children with mental health disabilities, these dynamics are particularly salient given the moral scrutiny often placed on parenting practices and the enduring stigma associated with mental illness (Corrigan & Miller, 2004).

Building on Goffman's (1963) foundational conceptualization of stigma as a socially produced process of devaluation, Stewart et al. (2025) advance a multidimensional framework (see Pryor et al., 2012) that distinguishes four interrelated types of stigma experienced by parents of children with mental health disabilities: public stigma, courtesy stigma, self-stigma, and structural stigma. This framework extends prior stigma models by centering parents' lived experiences and by explicitly linking stigma processes to employment, service access, and family well-being across the life course.

Public stigma refers to widely held negative stereotypes and societal attitudes toward mental illness that frame children with mental health disabilities, and by extension their parents, as dangerous, incompetent, or morally suspect. Parents routinely encounter public stigma in schools, workplaces, and community settings where children's behavioral expressions of distress are highly visible and poorly accommodated (Hinshaw, 2005; Stewart et al., 2025). These encounters shape parents' expectations of judgment and exclusion and influence how they approach institutions when seeking support.

Courtesy stigma operates through association, whereby parents are blamed for their child's mental health condition or perceived as deficient caregivers. This form of stigma is particularly salient in childhood mental health contexts, where parental responsibility is often foregrounded in explanations of children's behavior (Brennan et al., 2016; Rosenzweig et al., 2011; Stewart et al., 2025). Courtesy stigma intensifies parents' emotional labor and can undermine their credibility when advocating for services or accommodations across systems.

Self-stigma reflects the internalization of public and courtesy stigma, shaping parents' self-perceptions, sense of efficacy, and willingness to seek help. Repeated exposure to stigmatizing responses can lead parents to normalize inequitable treatment or to question their own competence, further constraining engagement with formal supports (Stewart et al., 2025). Self-stigma thus functions as an intrapersonal mechanism through which broader social devaluation is reproduced over time.

Structural stigma refers to institutional policies, practices, and norms that systematically disadvantage families caring for children with mental health disabilities (Stewart et al., 2025). Examples include fragmented eligibility criteria, discretionary accommodations, inconsistent enforcement of legal protections, and service systems that require repeated disclosure to access support. Structural stigma is particularly consequential because it embeds *inequity* within routine organizational processes, making exclusion appear neutral or unavoidable.

Rolland's Family Adjustment to Chronic Illness model (1993) provides an essential family-systems framework for understanding how these stigma processes interact with illness-related characteristics such as timing of onset, course, uncertainty, and outcome expectations (Rolland, 1993, 2025). Mental health disabilities frequently follow episodic or relapsing courses, requiring families to repeatedly reorganize roles, routines, and expectations in response to alternating periods of crisis and stability. Stigma compounds this uncertainty by shaping how families interpret symptoms, anticipate institutional responses, and allocate emotional and practical resources over time (Stewart et al., 2018).

Border and boundary theory further clarifies how parents respond to stigmatized environments at the interactional level (Ashforth et al., 2000; Clark, 2000; Gates & Akabas, 2010). Figure 3.1 illustrates how parents engage in ongoing boundary work to manage disclosure, role permeability, and exposure to stigma across family, workplace, and community contexts in relation to their child's life course and illness transitions. Decisions about whether, when, and how to disclose a child's mental health needs are shaped by prior experiences of public, courtesy, and structural stigma, leading many parents to adopt selective or cautious disclosure strategies (Rosenzweig et al., 2011; Stewart & Charles, 2022; Stewart et al., 2025).

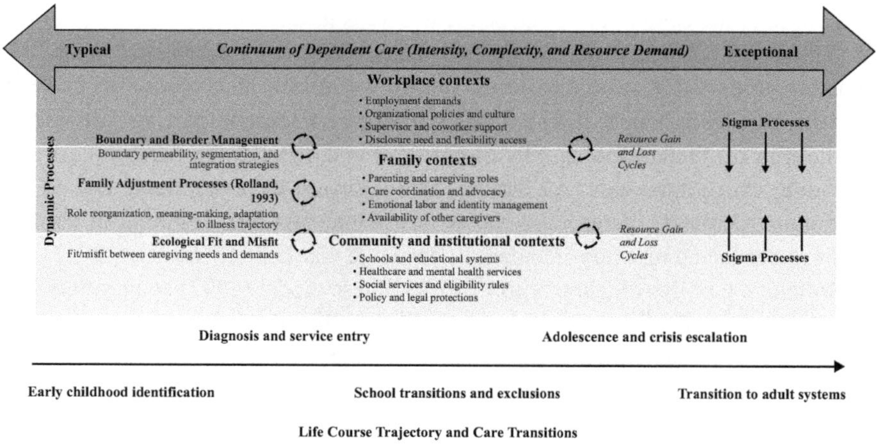

FIGURE 3.1 An Integrated Theoretical Model of Parenting a Child with a Mental Health Disability across Work, Family, and Community Contexts

Over time, repeated exposure to stigmatizing or inconsistent institutional responses shapes both family adaptation and boundary strategies. Parents may withdraw from formal systems, rely on increasingly narrow social networks, or disengage from employment or community participation when supports are unreliable or punitive. Empirical research documents how these processes contribute to social network contraction, caregiver isolation, and declining well-being among parents caring for children with mental health disabilities (Dembo et al., 2023). These patterns illustrate how stigma and structural barriers operate together to produce persistent ecological misfit across the life course.

Part 4: The Continuum of Dependent Care and the Dynamics of Work–Family Fit

The Continuum of Dependent Care model was developed to address limitations in traditional work–family and caregiving frameworks that assume caregiving demands are predictable, time-limited, and developmentally normative and that disability related care was a form of more intense caring (Stewart et al., 2018). While these assumptions may hold for typical caregiving trajectories, they fail to capture the intensity, complexity, and volatility of care demands experienced by parents of children with mental health disabilities.

The model conceptualizes dependent care along a continuum, with typical care on one end and exceptional care on the other. Movement along the continuum is not linear or unidirectional. Instead, families shift along the continuum in response to changes in care intensity, typology, complexity, and resource availability (Stewart et al., 2018). For parents of children with mental health disabilities, these shifts are often abrupt and recurrent, reflecting the episodic and crisis-driven nature of many psychiatric conditions.

Central to the Continuum of Dependent Care is its alignment with work–family fit (Voydanoff, 2005). Work–family fit is achieved when a parent's roles are adequately supported by resources across family, workplace, and community systems (Voydanoff, 2005; Moen, 2011). The Continuum of Dependent Care provides a mechanism for understanding why fit is fragile and difficult to sustain for parents providing exceptional care. As families move toward the exceptional end of the continuum, demands increasingly exceed available supports, resulting in chronic misfit rather than temporary imbalance (Brown & Clark, 2017; Stewart, 2013).

Rolland's Family Adjustment to Chronic Illness model (1993) again offers further explanatory depth by clarifying how illness characteristics shape movement along the continuum (Rolland, 1993; Rolland, 2025). Mental health disabilities are frequently characterized by *onset*, *uncertain prognosis*, and r*elapsing* or *episodic* courses. These features require families to repeatedly reorganize roles, routines, and expectations, often during key developmental transitions. When illness-related demands coincide with periods of reduced institutional support, such as school transitions or adolescence, families are pushed further toward the exceptional end of the continuum. Boundary and border theories as discussed in Part 2 above explain how parents attempt to manage these escalating demands in pursuit of work–family fit (Ashforth et al., 2000; Clark, 2000; Gates & Akabas, 2010). Stigma functions as a powerful force shaping movement along the continuum. Public, courtesy, self, and structural stigma influence not only how parents are perceived but how resources are accessed and sustained over time (Stewart et al., 2025).

Over time, persistent misfit along the Continuum of Dependent Care has cumulative consequences for parental health, employment stability, and social participation. Empirical research demonstrates that parents providing exceptional care to a child with a disability including a mental health need are more likely to experience work disruptions, income instability, sleep problems, and deteriorating physical and mental health compared to parents providing typical care (Sellmaier, 2021; Sellmaier et al., 2018, 2020, 2022). Social networks may contract as families exhaust informal supports, further reducing their capacity to absorb future care demands (Dembo et al., 2023).

As illustrated in Figure 3.1, the Continuum of Dependent Care integrates life course timing, family adjustment processes, boundary management, stigma, and ecological fit into a single explanatory framework. Rather than viewing caregiving challenges as isolated stressors or individual coping failures, the model highlights how structural conditions and disability-specific demands shape families' capacity to achieve and sustain work–family fit. For social workers, the Continuum of Dependent Care provides a conceptual tool for assessing caregiving demands, identifying points of intervention, and advocating for policies and organizational practices that recognize exceptional care as a shared social responsibility.

Part 5: Twenty Years of Research on Parenting, Work, and Community—Clarifying Key Drivers of Fit and Misfit

Over the past two decades, a sustained and collaborative body of research led by a small group of disability and social work scholars has reshaped how social work and allied disciplines understand the intersection of parenting, employment, and community life for families raising children with mental health disabilities. Collectively, this scholarship has demonstrated that disability-related caregiving introduces qualitatively different demands than typical parenting, requiring distinct theoretical frameworks that account for crisis-driven care, stigma, and structural constraint. Rather than treating work–family conflict as a universal experience, this body of work has clarified how parents' capacity to achieve and sustain work–family fit is shaped by the interaction of workplace and community systems over time.

Early Empirical Foundations: Exceptional Care as a Distinct Work–Family Condition

Early studies by Brennan, Rosenzweig, and colleagues disrupted dominant assumptions that work–family conflict functions similarly across families. Using qualitative and survey-based research, Brannan and Heflinger (2006), Rosenzweig et al. (2002), and Brennan et al. (2007) documented that parents of children with emotional and behavioral disorders experienced chronic employment disruption driven by crisis response, service coordination, and school-related demands. These findings established exceptional care as a persistent work–family condition rather than a temporary stressor, laying the groundwork for subsequent theoretical and policy developments. Building on this foundation, Rosenzweig et al. (2002) and Stewart (2013) demonstrated that parents providing exceptional care experienced elevated and sustained levels of both work–family and family–work conflict compared to parents providing typical care. Importantly, these studies showed that conventional workplace supports were often insufficient in the face of unpredictable caregiving demands, highlighting the need for frameworks that moved beyond time-based conflict to examine fit, flexibility, and structural responsiveness.

Gender, Family Structure, and Employment Constraint

A parallel line of research examined how caregiving demands intersect with gendered labor markets and family structure. DeRigne and Porterfield (2010, 2017) provided compelling evidence that mothers of children with disabilities were significantly more likely to reduce work hours or exit the labor force, particularly when access to coordinated services was limited. Their work reframed labor force withdrawal not as a matter of choice but as a structurally constrained outcome shaped by caregiving intensity and policy gaps. Sellmaier's (2019a; 2019b; 2022) work on fathers showed that even if fathers did not reduce their hours or gave up employment, they made employment decisions to better align work and care responsibilities. For example, they conducted extensive research about a job's benefits package before applying or they declined promotions that would have required extensive travel. These findings were confirmed by Stewart et al. (2013; 2024) and Sellmaier et al. (2016, 2020a, 2020b), who demonstrated that employment decisions among parents of children with mental health disabilities were driven by caregiving complexity, symptom severity, and time spent coordinating care. Together, this research underscored that gendered employment patterns among these families reflect unequal access to supports rather than differences in commitment or preference.

Workplace Systems: Fit, Disclosure, and Stigma

A central contribution of this research program has been the identification of workplace systems as a critical determinant of parental well-being and employment stability. Stewart's work has been particularly influential in theorizing how work–family fit is shaped by organizational culture, supervisor support, job autonomy, and access to flexibility (Stewart, 2013; Stewart et al., 2018, 2022). These studies demonstrated that when workplace supports aligned with caregiving demands, parents were better able to maintain employment and protect their health, even under conditions of exceptional care. However, this work also revealed that access to workplace support is often contingent on disclosure, exposing parents to stigma and discrimination. Rosenzweig et al. (2011) and Brennan et al. (2016) introduced the concept of courtesy stigma into the work–family literature, showing how parents were penalized for caregiving-related interruptions and labeled as both inadequate employees and deficient parents. Stewart and Charles (2022) extended this work by confirming disclosure of a stigmatized identity as a form of boundary management shaped by prior institutional encounters and that the stigma experienced was separate than flexibility stigma by workers with other types of caregiving. Their findings illustrated how parents developed increasingly cautious disclosure strategies over time, often concealing caregiving needs to preserve job security, even when formal supports were available.

Community Context: Services, Coordination, and Resilience

Complementing the focus on workplace systems, Sellmaier's scholarship has foregrounded the role of community context in shaping family adaptation and resilience under exceptional care demands. Her work has demonstrated that access to coordinated community services, supportive neighborhoods, and informal social networks can buffer stress and support caregiving capacity, even when workplace supports are limited (Sellmaier, 2019a; 2019b; Sellmaier et al., 2020a). Conversely, fragmented service systems, long waitlists, and inequitable access to care can intensify caregiving demands and undermine parents' ability to remain employed. Sellmaier's work also contributes a strengths-based perspective, highlighting how families cultivate resilience and meaning-making within constrained community environments. This focus on community-level resources and adaptive processes complements workplace-focused analyses by demonstrating that work–family fit cannot be achieved through employment interventions alone when community systems fail to meet families' needs. We will further discuss the impact of community resources in Chapter 6.

Health, Resources, and Cumulative Consequences

As this research program matured, attention increasingly turned to the cumulative consequences of persistent work–family misfit for parental health and well-being. Using national datasets, Stewart et al. (2018, 2022, 2024) and Sellmaier (2021) demonstrated that parents providing exceptional care reported poorer sleep, worse physical health, and higher stress than parents providing typical care. Organizational support and job autonomy emerged as protective factors, yet access to these resources remained uneven and often constrained by stigma and disclosure risk. More recent studies further documented how structural factors such as immigration status, neighborhood safety, and access to coordinated services shape parents' employment trajectories (Stewart et al., 2024; Sellmaier et al., 2020).

Integrating Theory and Evidence: From Description to Action

Together, this 20-year body of research provides a robust empirical foundation for the theoretical frameworks advanced in this chapter. It demonstrates that parenting a child with a mental health disability is shaped by the interaction of workplace systems, community context, stigma processes, and caregiving intensity across the life course. When disability-specific variables such as exceptional care demands, boundary management, courtesy stigma, and ecological resource fit are incorporated into work–family models, key drivers of parental well-being become visible. This integrated evidence base underpins the Continuum of Dependent Care model and supports the shift from deficit-based interpretations of caregiving toward a fit-based, systems-oriented approach. For social workers, these findings underscore the importance of interventions that simultaneously address workplace practices, community service coordination, and stigma reduction. For policymakers and organizations, they highlight the need for reforms that recognize caregiving as a shared social responsibility rather than an individual burden.

Table 3.2 translates these frameworks into actionable strategies for social work assessment, intervention, and policy practice. It illustrates how each theory informs practice decisions across micro, mezzo, and macro levels when supporting parents of children with mental health disabilities.

Part 6: Summary and Key Points

This chapter demonstrates that theoretical frameworks drawn from life course, boundary and border, ecological systems, family systems, and disability studies offer a robust foundation for understanding how parents navigate the uncertainty of raising a child with a mental health disability. Together, these perspectives illuminate how caregiving unfolds over time in unpredictable ways, how parents continually negotiate boundaries between work, family, and community life, and how stigma, organizational practices, and structural conditions shape parents' well-being and capacity to care.

For social work practice, this synthesis highlights the importance of centering parents' lived experiences as they navigate fragmented systems, shifting caregiving demands, and high-stakes decisions about disclosure, employment, and service access. Social workers are uniquely positioned to recognize how parents seek, lose, and regain work–family fit under conditions of uncertainty, and to advocate for integrated care systems, family-supportive workplaces, and stigma-informed responses that reduce isolation rather than exacerbate it.

Taken together, the theories outlined in this chapter provide a conceptual roadmap for supporting parents as they navigate the unknown. By treating caregiving as a shared social responsibility rather than an individual burden, social work can help transform uncertainty from a source of chronic strain into an organizing principle for responsive, coordinated, and equitable systems of support across the life course.

TABLE 3.2 Practice Integration Summary: Translating Theory into Social Work Assessment, Intervention, and Policy Action

Theoretical framework	*Practice focus*	*Assessment tools or approaches*	*Intervention strategies*	*Policy and Systems Levers*
Life Course Theory (Elder, 1998)	Anticipating family transitions and cumulative stress across time	• Life course mapping • Family timeline interviews • Caregiving trajectory assessment	• Transitional planning and anticipatory guidance during major milestones (e.g., school transitions, adolescence) • Strength-based life narrative work	• Advocate for lifespan and developmental flexibility in service eligibility (e.g., IDEA reauthorization, parental leave extensions)
Border/Boundary Theory (Clark, 2000)	Navigating work–family boundaries and disclosure decisions	• Work–family fit surveys (e.g., Voydanoff Scales) • Disclosure Decision-Making Aid (Stewart & Charles, 2022)	• Coaching for boundary negotiation and communication competence • Supervisor training in family-supportive leadership	• Workplace legislation promoting flexible scheduling and anti-discrimination protections (e.g., caregiver status as protected class)
Ecological Systems / Ecological Fit Theory (Bronfenbrenner, 1979; Voydanoff, 2005)	Assessing alignment between family needs and systemic supports	• Eco-map and genogram with community resource overlay • Family Needs Scale or Family Resource Scale (Brannan et al., 2006)	• Case management using coordinated care teams • Interdisciplinary service planning with schools and employers	• Promote integrated care models (e.g., wraparound, systems of care initiatives) and equitable access to behavioral health resources
Family Systems–Illness Model (Rolland, 1993)	Understanding family adaptation to chronic mental health conditions	• Family Adaptation and Cohesion Evaluation Scales (FACES-IV) • Family Meaning-Making Interviews	• Family psychoeducation on illness trajectory • Narrative reconstruction interventions • Family therapy emphasizing relational flexibility	• Expand reimbursement for family therapy and caregiver participation in treatment planning • Integrate family-centered outcomes in children's mental health policy

(*Continued*)

TABLE 3.2 (Continued)

Theoretical framework	*Practice focus*	*Assessment tools or approaches*	*Intervention strategies*	*Policy and Systems Levers*
Stigma Theory (Goffman, 1963)	Addressing felt, enacted, and structural stigma in family and work contexts	• Stigma Impact Scale	• Stigma-informed practice training • Peer support and empowerment groups for parents • Employer education to reduce courtesy stigma	• Anti-stigma public campaigns; inclusion of parents and caregivers in mental health equity legislation
Continuum of Dependent Care Model (Stewart et al., 2018)	Assessing intensity and complexity of caregiving demands	• Caregiver Strain Index (Brannan & Heflinger, 2006) • Caregiving Intensity Scale adapted for parents of children with mental health needs	• Tailor interventions according to level of caregiving intensity • Link high-intensity caregivers with respite and wraparound services	• Expand family leave policies to include episodic and cyclical caregiving • Develop funding streams for caregiver navigation and coordination supports
Conservation of Resources Theory (COR) (Hobfoll, 2011; Stewart et al., 2022)	Evaluating resource loss and gain cycles influencing stress and health	• Resource Assessment Matrix • Perceived Stress Scale • Work–Family Resource Fit Inventory	• Resource-building interventions (respite, flexible work, peer mentorship) • Wellness and sleep interventions for caregiver health	• Workplace and community wellness initiatives • Federal and provincial caregiver tax credits or stipends to offset resource depletion

Part 7: Application for Social Work Education

CASE VIGNETTE: A SOCIAL WORK CASE ILLUSTRATION OF APPLYING THE THEORETICAL FRAMEWORKS IN PRACTICE

Competency 6: Engage with Individuals, Families, Groups, Organizations, and Communities

Competency 7: Assess Individuals, Families, Groups, Organizations, and Communities

Competency 8: Intervene with Individuals, Families, Groups, Organizations, and

Learning outcomes

After engaging with this case vignette, students will be able to:

1. Apply multiple theoretical frameworks (life course, boundary, ecological systems, family systems, stigma, conservation of resources, and the Continuum of Dependent Care) to assess the experiences of parents raising children with mental health disabilities across work, family, and community contexts.
2. Analyze caregiving demands using a systems lens, identifying how micro-level stressors intersect with mezzo-level organizational practices and macro-level policy structures to shape family well-being and employment stability.
3. Demonstrate theory-informed intervention planning by identifying appropriate strategies at the individual, organizational, and policy levels that promote work–family fit, reduce stigma, and prevent caregiver resource depletion.
4. Evaluate the role of stigma and disclosure in shaping parental decision-making and employment outcomes, and articulate strategies for stigma-informed and rights-based social work practice.
5. Integrate assessment of care intensity and resource fit using the Continuum of Dependent Care Model to align supports with caregiving complexity rather than relying on deficit-based interpretations of parental functioning.
6. Articulate the role of social workers as boundary spanners and advocates, coordinating across systems and advancing structural change that recognizes caregiving as a shared social responsibility.

Case background

Maria is a 39-year-old single mother working full time as a medical assistant in a community health clinic. Her 12-year-old son, Jordan, has recently been diagnosed with generalized anxiety disorder and attention-deficit/

hyperactivity disorder (ADHD). Over the past year, Jordan's symptoms have worsened, leading to frequent calls from school, disciplinary suspensions, and missed workdays for Maria. She is exhausted, worried about losing her job, and reluctant to tell her supervisor about Jordan's diagnosis. When she is referred to a hospital-based family social worker for support, the social worker applies multiple theoretical frameworks to understand and intervene within Maria's overlapping systems of stress, responsibility, and care.

Life Course Theory: Identifying Turning Points and Transitions

Drawing on Elder's (1998) life course theory, the social worker begins by mapping the family's trajectory. She helps Maria reflect on key transitions, Jordan's move into middle school, the onset of behavioral changes, and the recent mental health diagnosis, as critical turning points that disrupt the family's stability. This lens positions Maria not as a "noncompliant parent" but as a caregiver navigating a developmental crisis within a broader family life course. The social worker uses this insight to develop an *anticipatory care plan*, preparing for upcoming transitions such as adolescence and high school entry. At the *micro level*, this helps Maria plan ahead; at the *macro level*, it underscores the importance of continuity in school and mental health supports over time.

Boundary Theory: Managing Work–Family Integration and Disclosure

Using Clark's (2000) *border theory*, the social worker explores Maria's struggle to separate her work and home roles. Maria feels guilty leaving work early but fears being labeled unreliable if she discloses Jordan's needs. Through coaching, the social worker helps her evaluate the risks and benefits of disclosure and to plan a targeted conversation with her supervisor using the *myChoice Disclosure Decision Aid.* At the *mezzo level*, the social worker connects with Maria's workplace employee assistance program to ensure that her request for modified scheduling is supported within organizational policy. This approach validates Maria's right to manage caregiving boundaries without stigma while maintaining employment stability.

Ecological systems Theory: Strengthening Interconnected Supports

The social worker creates an eco-map to visualize how Maria's microsystem (family, workplace, school) interacts with her mesosystem (community services, health care, and after-school programs). She identifies service gaps, limited coordination between Jordan's school counselor and his community therapist and facilitates a cross-system case conference to align support plans. This intervention draws directly on Voydanoff's (2005) adaptation of Bronfenbrenner's ecological theory, emphasizing the importance of fit between family demands and available resources. At the *macro level,* the case conference reveals a lack of system integration typical for families of children with mental health disabilities, reinforcing the need for policy-level advocacy for coordinated care.

Family systems–Illness Model: Understanding Family Adaptation

Applying Rolland's (1993) Family Systems–Illness Model, the social worker explores how Jordan's diagnosis affects the family's emotional climate and communication patterns. Maria initially sees the diagnosis as a personal failure. Through narrative reframing and psychoeducation, the social worker helps her construct a new meaning: that Jordan's anxiety is a treatable condition, not a reflection of poor parenting. This process restores family cohesion and strengthens Maria's sense of competence. At the *micro level*, the intervention builds resilience through shared understanding; at the *mezzo level*, it provides a framework for engaging extended family members as supports.

Stigma Theory: Addressing Courtesy and Structural Stigma

Maria's reluctance to discuss Jordan's condition at work reflects *courtesy stigma*, the fear of being devalued because of her child's mental health needs (Goffman, 1963; Stewart et al., 2025). The social worker validates her experience, normalizing stigma as a systemic issue rather than an individual weakness. Together, they develop strategies for selective disclosure and peer support engagement. At the *mezzo level*, the social worker collaborates with the clinic's human resources department to suggest an anti-stigma training module for managers, aligning with organizational diversity and inclusion goals. This dual approach reduces personal shame while challenging structural discrimination.

Continuum of dependent Care Model: Assessing Care Intensity and Resource Fit

To better understand Maria's situation, the social worker uses the Continuum of Dependent Care Model (Stewart et al., 2018). This framework places Maria's caregiving demands on the "exceptional care" end of the continuum due to the chronic, unpredictable, and emotional nature of Jordan's needs. The social worker helps Maria inventory her available resources, flexible work hours, family support, coping capacity and identify gaps. Recognizing that Maria's care intensity exceeds her resource capacity, the social worker advocates for additional community-based respite services and family navigation support. She and Maria also discuss whether Maria should disclose to her employer her child's care needs as a way of gaining workplace support. This application of the continuum model aligns resource allocation with caregiving complexity, moving from a deficit lens to a *fit* lens.

Conservation of Resources Theory: Preventing Resource Depletion

Finally, the social worker applies Hobfoll's (2011) Conservation of Resources theory, recognizing that Maria's chronic fatigue, financial strain, and emotional depletion stem from ongoing resource loss. The intervention focuses on stabilizing resource flows, connecting her with a caregiver support group, facilitating access to paid time off, and helping her apply for a local grant that offsets child therapy costs. At the macro level, the social worker documents Maria's experience to contribute to agency advocacy efforts aimed at expanding caregiver financial supports.

Integrative Practice across Levels

Over six months, Maria experiences tangible improvement: she negotiates a flexible schedule, Jordan's school implements accommodations, and family stress decreases. This case demonstrates how integrating multiple frameworks allows social workers to move fluidly between micro (individual and family), mezzo (workplace and community systems), and macro (policy and advocacy) levels of practice.

Micro: Assessment and intervention emphasize coping, boundary management, and meaning-making.

Mezzo: System coordination and workplace engagement address stigma and structural barriers.

Macro: Documentation and policy advocacy advance inclusive employment and mental health policy.

By grounding practice in these interconnected theories, social workers can recognize that parental well-being is shaped not only by individual resilience but by the interplay of resources, systems, and stigma. The goal is not simply to help families cope but to transform the environments in which they live and work—creating workplaces, schools, and communities that recognize caregiving as a collective social responsibility.

Discussion Questions

1 Which theories discussed in this chapter are most helpful for understanding Maria's experiences as a parent and employee? Explain how at least two theories help you make sense of her caregiving challenges.
2 What key transitions or turning points are shaping Maria and Jordan's current situation? How might these transitions affect the family over time?
3 Why is Maria hesitant to disclose her child's mental health needs at work? How can boundary theory and stigma theory help explain her concerns, and how might a decision aid like *myChoice* support her decision-making?

4 Where do you see gaps or mismatches between Maria's caregiving demands and the supports available to her? Identify one strategy at the individual, organizational, or policy level that could improve support for this family.
5 How does reframing Jordan's diagnosis help reduce Maria's feelings of guilt and strengthen family resilience? Why is this an important part of social work practice?
6 What lessons from Maria's case could inform changes in workplaces, schools, or policies that affect families raising children with mental health disabilities?

Resource List

Elder, G. H., Jr., Shanahan, M. J., & Jennings, J. A. (2015). Human development in time and place. In M. H. Bornstein, T. Leventhal, & R. M. Lerner (Eds.), *Handbook of child psychology and developmental science: Ecological settings and processes* (7th ed., pp. 6–54). John Wiley & Sons, Inc. https://doi.org/10.1002/9781118963418.childpsy402

Rolland, J. S. (2025). Chronic Illness and Disability: A Multisystemic Practice Model. *Journal of Family Nursing*, 31(2):63–74. doi:10.1177/10748407251329694

Rosenzweig J. M., & Brennan, E. M. (2008), *Work, life, and the mental health system of care: A guide for professionals supporting families of children with emotional or behavioral disorders*. Baltimore, MD: Paul H. Brookes.

Voydanoff, P. (2005). *Work, family, and community: Exploring interconnections.* Lawrence Erlbaum Associates.

References

Ashforth, B. E., Kreiner, G. E., & Fugate, M. (2000). All in a day's work: Boundaries and micro role transitions. *Academy of Management Review*, *25*(3), 472–491. https://www.jstor.org/stable/259305

Bitsko, R. H. (2022). Mental Health Surveillance Among Children—United States, 2013–2019. *MMWR Supplements*, 71. https://doi.org/10.15585/mmwr.su7102a1

Bitsko, R. H., Holbrook, J. R., Robinson, L. R., Kaminski, J. W., Ghandour, R., Smith, C., & Peacock, G. (2016). Health care, family, and community factors associated with mental, behavioral, and developmental disorders in early childhood—United States, 2011–2012. *MMWR. Morbidity and Mortality Weekly Report*, *65*(9), 221–226. https://doi.org/10.15585/mmwr.mm6509a1

Brannan, A., Manteuffel, B., Wayne Holden, E. *et al.* (2006). Use of the family resource scale in children's mental health: Reliability and validity among economically diverse samples. *Adm Policy Ment Health*, *33*, 182–197 (2006). https://doi.org/10.1007/s10488-006-0032-8

Brannan, A. M., Brennan, E. M., Sellmaier, C., & Rosenzweig, J. M. (2018). Employed parents of children receiving mental health services: Caregiver strain and work-life integration. *Families in Society*, *99*(1), 29–44. https://doi.org/10.1177/1044389418756375

Brannan, A. M., Brennan, E. M., Sellmaier, C., & Rosenzweig, J. (2022). Factors contributing to employment status over time for caregivers of young people with mental health disorders. *Healthcare*, *10*(8), 1562–1578. http://doi.org/10.3390/healthcare10081562

Brannan, A. M., & Heflinger, C. A. (2006). Caregiver, child, family and service system contributors to caregiver strain in two child mental health service systems. *The Journal of Behavioral Health Services & Research, 33*(4), 408–422. https://doi.org/10.1007/s11414-006-9035-1

Brennan, E. M., Jivanjee, P., Rosenzweig, J. M., & Stewart, L. M. (2016). Challenges and supports for employed parents of children and youth with special needs. In T. Allen & L. Eby (Eds.), *Oxford Handbook of work and family* (pp. 165–181). New York: Oxford University Press.

Brennan, E. M., Rosenzweig, J. M., Huffstutter, K., & Ogilvie, A. (2007). Employed parents of children with mental health disorders: Workplace experiences and policy implications. *Families in Society, 88*(3), 399–408. https://doi.org/10.1606/1044-3894.3598

Bronfenbrenner, U. (1979). *The ecology of human development: Experiments by nature and design*. Harvard University Press.

Brown, T., & Clark, C. (2017). Parents of children with mental health disabilities and employment challenges: A review. *Community, Work & Family, 20*(3), 327–345. https://doi.org/10.1007/s10566-017-9407-0

Clark, S. C. (2000). Work/family border theory: A new theory of work/family balance. *Human Relations, 53*(6), 747–770. https://doi.org/10.1177/0018726700536001

Corrigan, P. W., & Miller, F. E. (2004). Shame, blame, and contamination: A review of the impact of mental illness stigma on family members. *Journal of Mental Health, 13*(6), 537–548. https://doi.org/10.1080/09638230400017004

Dembo, R. S., Mailick, M. R., Rudolph, A. E., Huntington, N., DaWalt, L. S., & Mitra, M. (2023). Social network diversity and mental health among mothers of individuals with autism. *American Journal on Intellectual and Developmental Disabilities, 128*(2), 101–118. https://doi.org/10.1352/1944-7558-128.2.101

DeRigne, L. A., & Porterfield, S. L. (2010). Employment change and the role of the medical home for married and single-mother families with children with special health care needs. *Social Science & Medicine, 70*, 631–641. https://doi.org/10.1016/j.socscimed.2009.10.054

DeRigne, L. A., & Porterfield, S. L. (2017). Employment change among married parents of children with special health care needs. *Journal of Family Issues*, (38), 579–606. https://doi.org/10.1177/0192513X15572368

Elder, G. H. (1998). The life course as developmental theory. *Child Development, 69*(1), 1–12. https://www.jstor.org/stable/1132065

Gates, L. B., & Akabas, S. H. (2010). *Workplace supports for parents of children with asthma*. The 14th Annual Conference of the Society for Social Work Research. https://sswr.confex.com/sswr/2010/webprogram/Paper12557.html

Goffman, E. (1963). *Stigma: Notes on the management of spoiled identity*. Prentice Hall.

Greenhaus, J. H., & Beutell, N. J. (1985). Sources of conflict between work and family roles. *Academy of Management Review, 10*, 76–88. https://doi.org/10.5465/amr.1985.4277352

Hinshaw, S. P. (2005). The stigmatization of mental illness in children and parents: Developmental issues, family concerns, and research needs. *Journal of Child Psychology and Psychiatry, 46*(7), 714–734. https://doi.org/10.1111/j.1469-7610.2005.01456.x

Hobfoll, S. E. (2011). Conservation of resources theory: Implications for stress, health, and resilience. In S. Folkman (Ed.), *The Oxford handbook of stress, health, and coping* (pp. 127–147). Oxford University Press.

Kossek, E. E., Perrigino, M. B., & Lautsch, B. A. (2022). Work-life flexibility policies from a boundary control and implementation perspective: A review and research framework. *Journal of Management, 49*(6), 2062–2108. https://doi.org/10.1177/01492063221140354

Kossek, E. E., & Thompson, R. (2016). Workplace flexibility: Integrating employer and employee perspectives to close the research-practice implementation gap. In T. Allen & L. T. Eby (Eds.), *Oxford Handbook of work and family* (pp. 255–270). Oxford University Press.

Liegghio, M. (2017). 'Not a good person': Family stigma of mental illness from the perspectives of young siblings. *Child & Family Social Work, 22*, 1237–1245. https://doi.org/10.1111/cfs.12340

Moen, P. (2011). From 'work–family' to the 'gendered life course' and 'fit': Five challenges to the field. *Community, Work & Family,* 14, 89–96.

Namkung, E. H., Song, J., Greenberg, J. S., & Mailick, M. R. (2015). The relative risk of divorce in parents of children with developmental disabilities. *Journal of Family Psychology, 29*(3), 359–368. https://doi.org/10.1352/1944-7558-120.6.514

Pleck, J. H. (1997). Paternal involvement: Levels, sources, and consequences. In: *The role of the father in child development (3rd ed.;* pp. 66–103). John Wiley & Sons, Inc.

Pryor, J. B., Reeder, G. D., & Monroe, A. E. (2012). The infection of bad company: Stigma by association. *Journal of Personality and Social Psychology, 102*(2), 224–241. https://doi.org/10.1037/a0026270

Rolland, J. S. (1993). *Families, illness, and disability: An integrative treatment model.* Basic Books.

Rolland, J. S. (2025). Chronic illness and disability: A multisystemic practice model. *Journal of Family Nursing, 31*(2), 63–74. https://doi.org/10.1177/10748407251329694

Rosenzweig, J. M., Barnett, R. C., Huffstutter, K. J., & Stewart, L.M. (2008). Work-life integration: History, theory, and strategy. In J. Rosenzweig & E. Brennan (Eds.), *Work, life, and the mental health system of care: A guide for professionals supporting families of children with emotional or behavioral disorders* (pp. 89–115). Baltimore, MD: Paul H. Brookes.

Rosenzweig, J. M., Brennan, E. M., & Ogilvie, A. (2002). Work-family fit: Voices of parents of children with emotional and behavioral disorders. *Social Work, 47*, 415–424. https://doi.org/10.1093/sw/47.4.415

Rosenzweig, J. M., Malsch, A. M., Brennan, E. M., Huffstutter, K. J., Stewart, L. M., & Lieberman, L. A. (2011). Managing communications at the work-life boundary: Parents of children and youth with mental health disorders and human resource professionals. *Best Practices in Mental Health: An International Journal, 7*(1), 67–93.

Roundtree, L., & Lynch, K. (2006). *Exploring the complexities of exceptional caregiving. Executive briefing series.* Boston College, Center for Work & Family.

Sellmaier, C. (2019a). Integrating work and family responsibilities: Experiences of fathers of children with special health care needs. *Journal of Child and Family Studies, 28*(11), 3022–3036. https://doi.org/10.1007/s10826-019-01478-6

Sellmaier, C. (2019b). Work, family, and community ecologies and their influence on work–life fit for fathers of children with special health care needs. *Families in Society: The Journal of Contemporary Social Services, 100*(1), 68–79. https://doi.org/10.1177/1044389418811945

Sellmaier, C. (2021). Physical and mental health of mothers and fathers caring for children with special health care needs: The influence of community resources. *Journal of Family Issues, 43*(11), 2815–2840. https://doi.org/10.1177/0192513X211035580

Sellmaier, C., & Buckingham, S. (2022). "I think sometimes that dads are kind of forgotten (…) so it's nice that we also get a voice.": Work-life experiences of employed U.S. fathers caring for a child with special health care needs. *Community, Work, & Family, 25*(5), 661–676. https://doi.org/10.1080/13668803.2021.1911935

Sellmaier, C., Leo, M. C., Brennan, E. M., Kendall, J., & Houck, G. M. (2016). Finding fit between work and family responsibilities when caring for children with ADHD diagnoses. *Journal of Child and Family Studies, 25*(12), 3684–3693. https://doi.org/10.1007/s10826-016-0527-1

Sellmaier, C., Stewart, L. M., Brennan, E. M., Rosenzweig, J. M., & Malsch, A. M. (2020a). Parents of children and youth with disabilities: Providing exceptional care and meeting work-life challenges. In S. A. Ammons (Ed.), *Work family encyclopedia.* Work-Family Researchers Network.

Sellmaier, C., Stewart, L. M., & Brennan, E. M. (2020b). Workforce engagement of children and youth with mental health disabilities: The impact of community services and supports. *Community, Work and Family*, *23*(5), 534–555. https://doi.org/10.1080/13668803.2020.1820954

Stewart, L. M. (2013). Family care responsibilities and employment: Exploring the impact of type of family care on work–family and family–work conflict. *Journal of Family Issues*, *34*(1), 113–138. https://doi.org/10.1177/0192513X12437708

Stewart, L. M., & Charles, A. (2022). To disclose or conceal? Workplace disability and eldercare-related disclosure decision-making strategies. *Journal of Family Issues*, *43*(6), 1536–1554. https://doi.org/10.1177/0192513X211026965

Stewart, L. M., Lile, W., & Stutz, H. (2018). The continuum of dependent family care: A theoretical explanation and model. *Special Issue Community, Work and Family*, *21*(5), 599–619. https://doi.org/doi:10.1080/13668803.2018.1530637

Stewart, L. M., Sellmaier, C., Brannan, A. M., & Brennan, E. M. (2022). Supporting sleep and health of employed parents with typical and exceptional care demands. *Journal of Social Service Research*, *48*(1), 1–17. https://doi.org/10.1080/01488376.2021.2024935

Stewart, L. M., Sellmaier, C., Henderson-Posther, M., Lukefahr, J., & Brennan, E. M. (2025). Navigating stigma and discrimination at work while parenting a child with a mental health disability. In *Disability and the family: Challenges, resources, and resilience* (Vol. 27, pp. 97–113). Emerald Publishing.

Stewart, L. M., Sellmaier, C., Shrestha, L., & Brennan, E. M. (2024). Factors influencing employment decisions among immigrants caring for a child with special health care needs. *Journal of Family Issues*, *45*(2), 394–418. https://doi.org/10.1177/0192513X221150981

Voydanoff, P. (2005). *Work, family, and community: Exploring interconnections*. Lawrence Erlbaum Associates.

4

THE FAMILY SYSTEM

This chapter will take a closer look at the impact of exceptional care responsibilities on the family system. We will first examine the effects on the parent individually and then dive into the marital or partner relationship. In addition, we will discuss how caring for a child with a mental health disability might affect sibling relationships and connections with extended family members. These conversations can often take a pathological view or problem focus. Aligned with our overall theoretical framework of a social model disability and a disability justice perspective, we added a section about family resilience both as an individual and as a social-ecological construct. At the beginning of each section, we included quotes from parents we interviewed over the years to exemplify the experiences of families.

Part 1: Effects of Exceptional Care on Parents Individually and on Their Relationship

> It's been a real strain on our marriage hm I mean financially ahm physically exhausted ahm because we have a division of labor we often don't know what the other one is up to sometimes and so when we ask questions we kind of take it personally ahm we're both taking sleeping pills to get to sleep because of the stress, it affected our sex life, it affected our ability to travel, self care, to recreate.

Receiving a medical diagnosis including a mental health diagnosis can be difficult for the individual and for the family and has been described as ambiguous. The ambiguity is a result of several factors including the lack of clarity of a diagnosis, unclear outcomes and long-term prospects, changes in well-being from day to day

DOI: 10.4324/9781003532668-4

and over time, as a hidden disability, the environment might not be aware of the disability and therefore might have unrealistic expectations, and a fear of disrupted family relationships. For example, parents describe receiving a diagnosis as an emotional rollercoaster moving between feelings of hopelessness and disbelief and hope and a sense of relief (Abbott et al., 2013; O'Brien, 2007). Especially if the path to a diagnosis was longer, parents felt some relief that there was a name to their worries at the same time causes of mental health issues are usually not clearly identifiable, and a treatment plan is usually not as well defined as treating a bacterial infection with antibiotics leaving parents with a great amount of uncertainty. Parents might also blame themselves for their child's mental health problems and question their competence as parents, in addition to grieving the loss of their dreams for the child's and the family's future (McCann et al., 2011; O'Brien, 2007). This loss can be described as ambiguous loss, which is defined as loss related to someone being either physically present but psychologically absent or being physically absent, but psychologically present (Boss, 1999). In the case of a mental health disability, the loved one is still physically present but might be psychologically absent. This overall ambiguity can increase family stress.

Caregiver strain, which is also discussed as caregiver burden or burden of care, measures the potential stress, responsibility, demands, and physical/psychological impact of caring for someone with a disability (Brannan et al., 1997). Brannan et al. (1997) distinguish between three areas of caregiver burden including objective caregiver strain, internalized subjective, and externalized subjective caregiver strain. Objective caregiver strain captures effects on physical and mental health, social, family, and community relationships, impacts on work and finances, and on personal time and family activities. Internalized subjective strain represents feelings of sadness, guilt, worry, and tiredness. Externalized subjective strain covers negative feelings toward the child such as anger, resentment, embarrassment, and strained relationship with the child. Caregiver strain illuminates the possibly complex and wide-ranging impact of exceptional care responsibilities on individual family members and the family system as a whole. The child's symptom levels appear to influence the level of strain experienced by parents, but access to resources plays a role as well. For example, parents who can meet their family's basic needs and report adequate housing seem to have less caregiver strain (Kvist et al., 2013) than parents struggling with meeting basic needs. Access to material resources can therefore have an effect on caregiver strain independent of the level of symptoms displayed by the child (McConnell et al., 2014).

It is also important to highlight that employment can be beneficial to caregivers independent or in addition to the material gains. Parents reported that going to work as a form of respite from caregiving and family responsibilities, a place to think about something else and to focus on one's own interests. Workplaces therefore can be an opportunity for parents to recharge (Lewis et al., 1999). This has been captured in quantitative research as positive work to family spillover (Grzywacz & Marks, 2000) (Figure 4.1). This is one dimension of the work-family

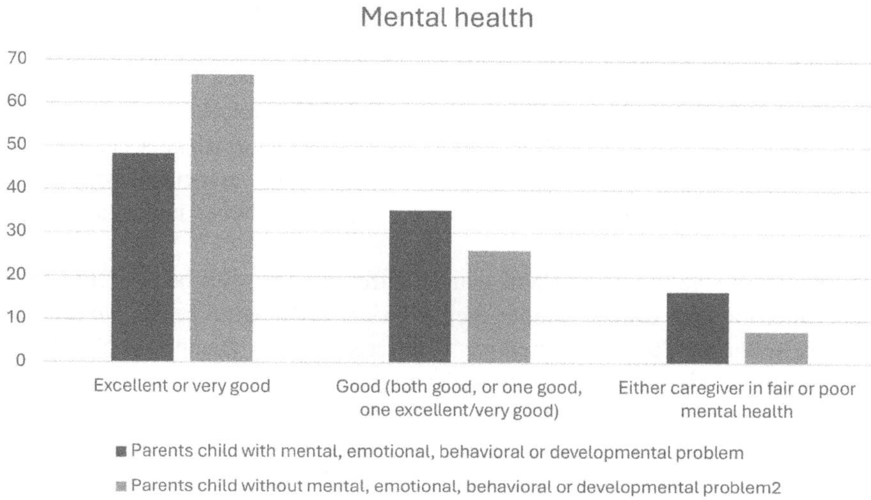

FIGURE 4.1 Mental Health Parents with and without Child with Mental Health Disability Based on Data from 2023/24 National Survey of Children's Health

interface, which also includes positive family to work, negative work to family, and negative family to work spillover. The potentially positive impact of work on family life includes job skills that are helpful at home or for solving personal issues, or work experiences making one a more interesting person or a better friend at home. Employment therefore can offer respite, positive experiences that provide a sense of agency and competence, and practical skills useful for problem-solving at home. One father I interviewed mentioned that his wife had social service experience, which was very helpful to understand what his son was going through, to provide information about the diagnosis, and to develop a service plan. He experienced his wife's professional experience as directly impactful to support his son and to lower some of the father's own stress (Sellmaier & Buckingham, 2022). This points to the importance of mental health services and treatment access for the well-being of the child and the family. If children receive services that reduce symptomology, then parents will also experience less caregiver strain (Brannan et al., 2018). In addition, service providers can offer social-emotional support to parents to adapt to the changes and to be able to deal more effectively with the ambiguity of the diagnosis, reducing overall levels of stress.

Differences in Experience

There are possible differences in the experience of stress to consider. For example, experiences of caregiver strain seem to differ based on race. Independent of a child's symptoms, African American parents reported less caregiver strain than White Non-Hispanic parents (Brannan et al., 2018; McCabe et al., 2003). In

McCabe et al.'s (2003) study, White Non-Hispanic parents reported the highest levels of caregiver strain compared to Latino, Asian Pacific Islander, and African American parents, although only the relationship between White and African American parents remained significant when accounting for child symptoms. Interestingly, in this study African American and Asian Pacific Islander parents also reported significantly less social support, which is usually associated with an increase in caregiver strain. Further research is needed to better understand these racial differences.

There is mixed evidence about gender differences in well-being. One study found that mothers evaluated both their physical and mental health worse than fathers (Sellmaier, 2021), which aligns with research from Brannan et al. (2018), which reported higher caregiver strain for mothers of children with mental health disabilities compared to fathers. Other studies did not find any differences in well-being between mothers and fathers (Ha et al., 2008).

Since mothers are still more likely to reduce work hours (Sellmaier et al., 2020) and to take on more of the care work (Sellmaier, 2019), they might experience less respite from care demands, which could impact their overall well-being and stress levels. It is critical to mention here that the majority of research is still focused on primary caregivers, which are more likely to be the mother. Our understanding of the experience of fathers is therefore still limited. My own research about fathers caring for a child with a disability found that fathers also struggle even though they were usually the main breadwinner and only had limited care responsibilities (Sellmaier, 2019; Sellmaier & Buckingham, 2022). Fathers reported trying to adjust their work schedule to be available for school drop offs, they

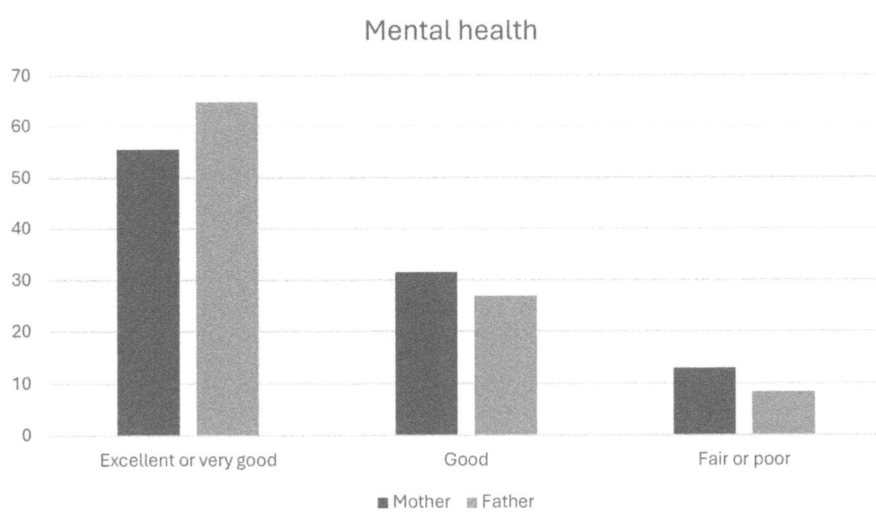

FIGURE 4.2 Mother and Father Mental Health Based on Data from 2023/2024 National Survey of Children's Health

declined opportunities for promotions if they would increase work travel, and they researched employment health insurance policies and state service delivery systems to make sure their children had access to needed treatments. Dads had these employment-related thoughts and considerations in addition to their worries about their children's futures, wondering if their children will be successful in school and if they should establish a trust fund for when they wouldn't be around anymore to care for them.

The Couple Relationship

Research about the impacts of raising a child with a disability on the parental relationship is mixed (Brown et al., 2020; Hartley et al., 2018; Kvist et al., 2013). For example, one Danish study showed that parents of children with ADHD diagnosis were more likely to get divorced or separate, but they also were more likely to have additional relationship stressors such as low socio-economic status, and their own mental health concerns (Kvist et al., 2013), which makes it more difficult to decipher if the child's diagnosis was the main driver for this increased divorce rate. This study also reported that the likelihood of divorce/separation went down once families had a diagnosis, since this probably allowed for access to treatment (Kvist et al., 2013). Uncertainty, unmanaged symptoms, and a lack of tools for parents and children might therefore be the more accurate description of the cause for increased relationship stressors, which is also reflected in the quote at the introduction of this chapter. Positive coping skills are therefore critical to deal with parenting stress and to improve marital satisfaction (Brown et al., 2020). Uncertainty about the diagnosis and about appropriate parenting strategies can also increase disagreements between couples on how to respond to certain behaviors, which can increase the risk for couple's conflict (Quittner et al., 1998). Most research about the impacts of exceptional care on a couple's relationship included heterosexual couples. A literature review on parenting stress and relationship quality between same-sex and different-sex parents in the general population did not find differences in either parenting stress or relationship quality. Although some studies found increased parenting stress due to experiences of discrimination (Jin & Mazrekaj, 2025). Further research should examine relationship quality specifically in same-sex couples caring for a child with a mental health disability. In addition to stressors related to care responsibilities, families are also more likely to struggle with integrating work and care demands, increasing work-family conflict (Stewart et al., 2023). Work-family conflict has been found to increase the risk for marital conflict (Minnotte et al., 2015). Every relationship is unique, but it is critical to keep in mind that exceptional care responsibilities specifically might affect the couple's relationship. Furthermore, the increased risk for work-family conflict and for economic insecurity due to the difficulties integrating work and care responsibilities and a lack of social services might also negatively affect the couple's relationship.

Part 2: Effects on Immediate and Extended Family Members

> Right now we can't just up and leave with our youngest son and the shape he is in we just can't leave him with anybody for a weekend or so because we because of some of his problems (…) I am hesitant to ask a lot of times but ah most people ah are willing to, you know, they do as much as they can.

> None of our family would be willing to provide respite they were scared that something medical would happen to my firstborn and then they were ahm really scared of my daughter's aggressive behaviors and so we were kind of on our own.

Overall, research demonstrates that families with exceptional care responsibilities are often dealing with social isolation and strained relationships with family members and the community at large (Friesen, 1989; Harden, 2005; Van Der Sanden et al., 2015). Parents have reported that extended family might stay away, since they struggle dealing with certain aspects of the child's disability, such as externalizing behaviors mentioned above. Families also reported that they might be more reluctant to plan or participate in activities outside the home, since they fear the reactions and stigmatization from others. Participants in our research reported that they were at times blamed for their child's mental health concerns (Sellmaier & Buckingham, 2022; Stewart et al., 2024). Blaming parenting as a cause for the disability seems more likely for mental health disabilities than for physical or intellectual disabilities. Mental health disabilities can also be understood as hidden disabilities, which seem to influence the public's response to certain behaviors. If a child has a visible disability, certain behaviors might be interpreted as appropriate, but if the child has a hidden disability, the behavior might be interpreted as inappropriate and the child or the parent be blamed as "bad." Age can play a role as well with the public perception being more lenient with younger than older children, as behavioral expectations grow with age. Parents reported experiencing this stigmatization in their communities and in their workplaces. Parents might also face a double bind being blamed for their child's disability and being targeted as "bad" employees (Stewart et al., 2024), which we discuss in greater detail in chapter 5. Fathers also talked about being asked why their spouse was not taking care of the child. This experience has been discussed in research as flexibility stigma, which more often targets male employees (Coltrane et al., 2013). Traditionally, men's role was conceptualized as the main breadwinner. Male employees who take time off or request flexibility to meet child care responsibilities are therefore not meeting societal expectations, which can lead to discrimination or stigmatization. For example, they might not be considered for promotions or might be assigned to less prestigious and influential projects.

Stigmatization and the reluctance of extended family members to deal with the child can be reasons for increased social isolation. Interestingly, our research has also found that families often moved to either find jobs that provided flexibility, much needed health care benefits, or better schools uprooting their social networks

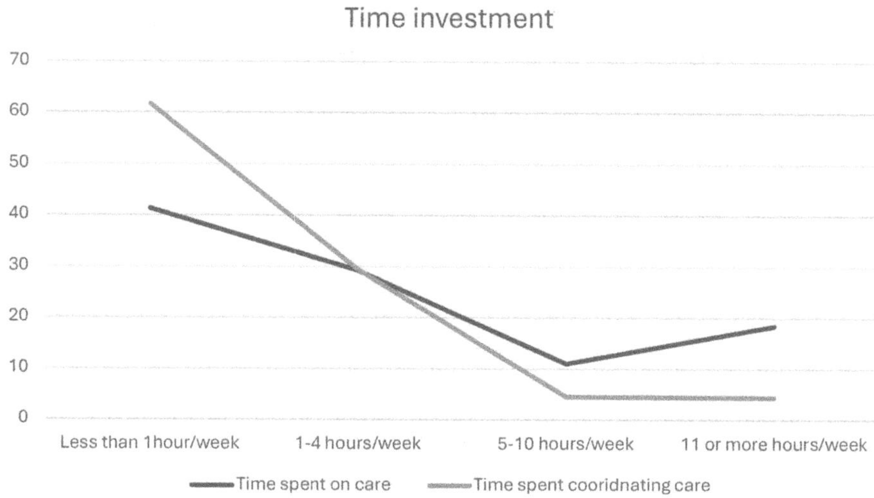

FIGURE 4.3 Time Caring and Coordinating Care Based on Data from 2023/2024 National Survey of Children's Health

and separating them from friends and extended family members (Sellmaier & Buckingham, 2022). Establishing new friendships and networks is always time-consuming which can be more difficult for families with exceptional care responsibilities. One common theme in our research has been that care responsibilities can be time intensive. One father shared that he goes to work and then goes home to help care for his children, leaving little to no time for leisure activities with his wife or friends (Sellmaier & Buckingham, 2022). Re-building social networks can therefore be challenging within the demands of exceptional care responsibilities.

Day-to-day experiences might also be quite different compared to parents who don't have exceptional care responsibilities making it more difficult to keep connections to existing friendships or to establishing new friendships. Peer-support networks can fill an important role here, since they provide a space to share experiences and to feel seen and understood by other caregivers with similar experiences. We will explore the relevance of peer-support in the later chapter on community resources. Strong social connections to family and friends are not just relevant to strengthen well-being and mental health, but it also provides instrumental support such as child care to maintain work or to have some respite from child care responsibilities.

Part 3: Effects on Sibling Relationships

Examining current research about siblings shows that the majority includes adult siblings (Levante et al., 2024), which includes issues that go beyond the scope of this book, such as decisions about providing care or financial support for the sibling (Barnable et al., 2006), but there are also some conclusions that are important to consider in the context of this book. Overall, the quality of the sibling relationship appears to be similar to relationships of siblings without disabilities, holding the potential for both positive and negative interactions (Levante et al., 2024). At the same time, there are some unique factors that warrant consideration. For example, siblings similar to parents, report dealing with shame and grief as they learn about their sibling's diagnosis. When siblings were diagnosed later in life, siblings mourned the loss of the previous relationship or the loss of their sibling as they used to be. Phases of grief aligned with Kübler-Ross' stages and included denial, anger, bargaining, depression, and relief (Riebschleger, 1991). These phases shouldn't be understood as a linear progression but as interconnected with siblings moving back and forth or skipping phases, especially if their sibling's symptoms were managed more or less well. As mentioned above, this grief has been described as ambiguous loss, since this loss of an imagined future or an imagined relationship is not acknowledged and mourned like death might be (Abrams, 2009). The stigma associated with mental illness further complicates the grieving process specifically and the sibling relationship more broadly, with the sibling being ashamed of their sibling's disability. They might then experience greater isolation, since they don't want to invite friends over for example. It also seems consistent across research (Abrams, 2009; Lively et al., 1995) that the time and energy that is required from parents to address one sibling's mental health needs leave the other child feeling neglected. Siblings might also be reluctant to reach out to parents if they are struggling because they don't want to be an additional burden for parents who are already stressed. Siblings might also feel guilty for being healthy. Some siblings reported becoming more focused in school and seeing school as an opportunity to be their own selves while others worked extra hard to make up for their siblings. Others also reported feeling distracted and worried and therefore struggling more in school (Lively et al., 1995). Considering this brief excursion on sibling relationships, we can summarize that siblings are affected by their sibling's mental health disability. How one is affected varies and depends on multiple factors. Services seem most focused on supporting the child with a diagnosis and when considering family impacts usually limit their attention to parents. It is therefore important to further examine the needs of siblings and develop specific supports for them.

Part 4: Family Resilience

> And it the one thing it does do so I will give it credit for this is that there are many times I am sitting in the board room or I am sitting in an executive meeting and everyone is freaking out over a problem and thinks it's such a huge deal. Yeah nobody's children are affected here nobody is has a life-altering decision it is just a problem we need to fix. Ahm, so it does give you having having children with special needs does give you some perspective on the rest of the world.

The previous sections discussed the stress potentially associated with raising a child with a mental health disability arguing that the whole family can be impacted. This discussion would be one-sided if we did not also talk about the possibility for growth available in difficult times. Walsh (2003) argues that family resilience is situated in the interaction of individual or family stressors and the family's social context. Ungar (2011) further explores this in his discussion of a social-ecological perspective on resilience, claiming that the environment and context are critical for thriving amidst uncertainty and stress. The focus is more heavily on the influence of micro, mezzo, and macro system factors than on individual characteristics or individual temperament. Ungar (2011) identified four aspects of this socio-ecological perspective of resilience including decentrality, complexity, atypicality, and cultural relativity. Decentrality argues that neither individual characteristics nor environmental factors adequately explain resilience, but that resilience is situated in the interplay between individual and environment. For example, individual characteristics such as hope and optimism can only act as protective factors in an environment that supports these traits. Environmental aspects have been identified as critical for thriving within adverse conditions. For example, supportive adults or economic stability improved outcomes of children and youth experiencing adversity. Another principle of resilience in this model is complexity. Ungar asserts that what makes someone more resilient be it individual or environmental factors are complex and change over time and in different environmental contexts. It is therefore difficult to identify factors that increase thriving for everyone all the time. Research seems to identify some patterns such as the protective nature of social connectedness, but even these patterns are complex and connected to a variety of other factors as well. Openness and not determinism are therefore warranted when assessing protective factors for individuals or families. Walsh (2003) also asserts that both crises and family systems develop and change requiring different adaptive responses at varying time points. The principle of complexity also ties into the principle of atypicality, challenging any notion that event A automatically leads to outcome B. This can also mean that certain behaviors are protective in certain environments even if they might be seen as problematic in the larger societal context. For example, disengaging emotionally from an abusive parent can reduce the stress experienced by the child. Understanding the context for certain behaviors can help better understand if these behaviors are productive or serve a larger function of dealing with difficult circumstances. The definition of resilience is also influenced by the individual's culture (Ungar, 2011) adding another layer of complexity and one model of family health does not fit all families (Walsh, 2003). In summary, resilience in this framework is understood as a process that shifts and changes and as highly contextual influenced by culture and the availability and accessibility of environmental resources that support thriving in stressful situations. Families with exceptional care responsibilities face challenges and their access and the availability of supportive resources is critical for resilience. Families are neither inherently resilient nor inherently non-resilient, but their ability to cope and thrive is influenced by their environmental context. Resilience is also not static, and families might be more or less resilient at different times. Resilience does not assume that families just return to the state they were in before a traumatic or challenging event, but Walsh (2003) describes this as springing forward allowing for a new organization and a re-structuring to successfully deal with the changes and challenges. Patterson (2002) integrated family stress and family resilience theories, developing a model that can also be helpful to understanding the challenges families face and the opportunities for thriving amidst these challenges. The Family Adjustment and Adaptation Response Model distinguishes between family adjustment and family adaptation. Families have access to certain resources or capabilities, and they must deal with certain demands. At times the demands might outpace the available capabilities. When families find ways to deal with these exceeding demands they exhibit successful adjustments. If this imbalance continues over time or if a family experiences a stressor that goes beyond the daily normative challenges and adjustment is impossible, families experience a crisis. In this crisis, families will either find ways to reduce demands, increase capabilities or change the meaning they associate with the crisis, potentially resulting in family adaptation. Patterson (2002) argues that family adaptation aligns with family resilience and that well adapted or resilient families can fulfill family functions. For example, families in our society are responsible for caring and raising their children and to support them economically. With limited financial support in the United States, maintaining employment while managing demanding care responsibilities demonstrates the resilience and adaptability of the family following Patterson's model. Supporting families' economic security can in this context be understood as supporting family resilience, providing an argument for the need to increase financial supports and workplace flexibility for families. The concept of positive family-to-work spillover is fitting as well. As mentioned above, families describe the positive effects of certain work skills and experiences on managing their family responsibilities. In the same way as work can positively affect our family lives, family experiences can also enhance our skillset at work. The quote at the beginning of this section is one example for this, since the father describes himself as more calm in stressful workplace situations due to his experiences caring for his sons, which makes him a more effective problem solver at work. Family responsibilities can make it more difficult to engage in work, but they can also be an asset and add to an employee's skillset. Unfortunately, we often don't highlight how our family experiences positively affect our work performance.

Similarly, parents being able to connect their children with mental health providers so they can receive treatment shows their resilience and their ability to meet the children's care needs. In this context, we can also consider a family's resources to meet the needs of siblings as discussed above. Additionally, well-supported parents with more effective coping skills show improved mental health and well-being independent of the child's level of care needs and symptoms (Bourke-Taylor et al., 2012; Churchill et al., 2010). Supporting the whole family should therefore

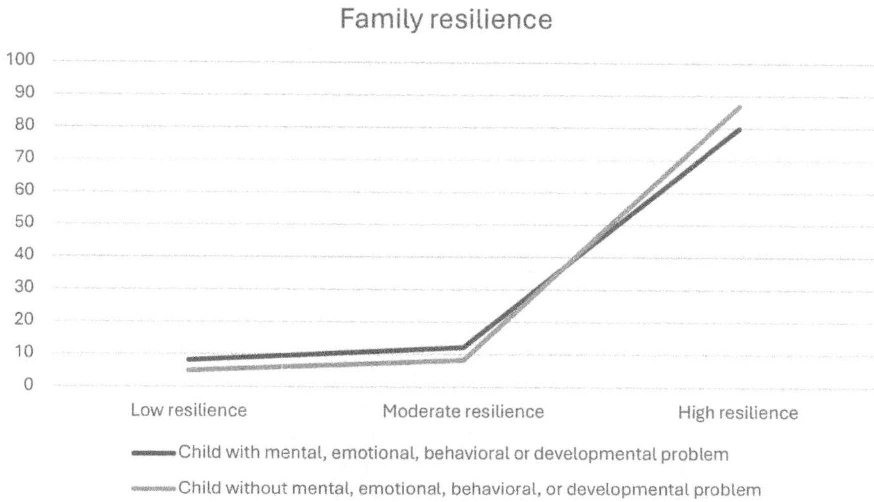

FIGURE 4.4 Family Resilience Based on Data from 2023/2024 National Survey of Children's Health

be standard practice. As Walsh (2006) argues in families especially with chronic health conditions, the illness or disability must be decentralized, and new routines have to be developed that bring all family members back into focus. The best timing for this work depends on the nature and stage of the condition and the family life cycle. First, families adjust to the new diagnosis or crisis and then long-term, they have to adapt to the chronic nature of illness and the often episodic nature of a mental health disability (Walsh, 2006). Family resilience is therefore not static but changes and varies over time as do the support needs of families.

Kendall and Shelton (2003) developed a model of four management styles of families with children with ADHD diagnoses based on interview data with 15 families, ranging from the chaotic, ADHD-controlled, surviving, and reinvested family. This study exemplifies the theoretical models introduced above, offering some specifics about how families might adapt to an ADHD diagnosis. Chaotic management styles refer to families who are extremely stressed who have access to very few resources and supports. In ADHD-controlled families, all family interactions are organized around ADHD symptomology, which can result in exhaustion, family conflict, and disengagement of some family members. Surviving families have re-focused their family life from disruptive symptoms to emotional and family well-being. This change in focus still comes at a high price, requiring great discipline and effort in parenting with limited outside support. The reinvested family was found to have accepted the child's disability and to have moved past guilt or attempts to "fix." They reinvested in their families, themselves, their work, and accepted ADHD as part of their family life without making it the center of their family life.

Part 5: Summary and Key Points

The whole family is affected if a child receives a mental health diagnosis. The care responsibilities, the worry about the future, or financial impacts can increase stress and strain for parents. Siblings also have to make sense of the diagnosis and the changes in the family often with little support from social service providers or parents who might be more focused on the child with the mental health disability. In addition, all family members might experience stigmatization due to the nature of the diagnosis and or might blame themselves for the child's mental health struggles. These challenges can put families into crisis mode straining their resources to successfully cope and adapt to the new and changing situation. Despite the reality of stress related to exceptional care experiences, families also adapt to change and thrive. Family resilience is an important component to consider both as a fact of family life and as a goal of interventions. Using a family resilience lens can help with assessing both the challenges and the resources and with applying a strength perspective instead of a deficit approach. As we will discuss in Chapters 5 and 6 specifically, the availability of workplace and community supports plays a critical role in mitigating family stress. The family experience therefore has to be considered not as an individual experience but as situated within the larger context of resources and policies.

- Caring for a child with a mental health disability affects the whole family system.
- There is an increased risk for stress, especially if workplace and community resources are inadequate or inaccessible.
- Families can thrive when they successfully adapt to the challenges and receive necessary community supports.

Part 6: Recommendations for Social Work Practice

Social workers, therapists, and service providers can play a crucial role in strengthening the whole family and support family resilience. Kendall and Shelton's study only included a small sample of families and was focused on children with ADHD, but the recommendations developed based on this examination seem relevant across diagnoses. For example, the authors suggest that chaotic families might first have to be stabilized in meeting their basic needs before social-emotional therapies can take place. If a family struggles to maintain housing, doesn't have access to stable child care or medical care, they are not well equipped to successfully deal with the demands of parenting a child with an ADHD diagnosis. Service providers should focus on stabilizing these families to free capacities for specific parenting techniques. In ADHD-controlled families who are exhausted from their all-consuming focus on the child with ADHD, a realignment of family energy and activity is warranted. Service providers who can step in as advocates and mentors for the child can relieve some of the burden felt by families. Family therapy can also help families to re-engage in fun activities, strengthening the positive family bonds. According to Kendall and Shelton's research, the surviving family would often receive the least support from service providers, because they appeared to be functional, advocating for their children, and implementing helpful parenting strategies. At the same time, these families were still struggling, often feeling overwhelmed and left alone by service providers. For these families, it is critical to receive an assessment from family members on how well things are going and what kind of supports they think are needed, since from the outside things might appear quite well-organized even though family members might still be struggling. The researchers noted that the children in reinvested families were all older, which might explain the level of management and re-alignment the families exposed. These families might need support with the transition of their children through adolescence and young adulthood when responsibilities shift from parents to children and the family dynamics change due to the family's life cycle. These examples highlight the need for individualized approaches to supporting families, since their needs likely vary due to the stage and nature of the diagnosis and the life stage of the family and the child. A resilience perspective also asks providers to assess family's strengths even in times of crises and assumes that every family has the capacity to thrive (Walsh, 2003).

Our own research about the importance of community resources for parental well-being and the works of our colleagues stress that family resilience includes economic resources and institutional supports such as flexible work schedules and access to health care (Brannan et al., 1997; Kendall & Shelton, 2003; Sellmaier, 2021; Walsh, 2003). Social workers who are interested in family resilience should therefore also engage in policy advocacy to realize paid family and medical leave for all families. An understanding of workplace rights and strategies to support parents navigating workplace policies and accessing workplace protections is required as well. Social workers still seem underrepresented in conversations about workplace policies and employment issues. Economic security is often focused on welfare policies, minimum wage discussions, or income tax credits. These are of course critical policies and issues, but they don't include strategies for families on how to handle exceptional care responsibilities in the workplace. For example, how to disclose challenging family situations with their supervisor to access flexibility or understanding their rights related to family responsibility discrimination. We will discuss the impact of policies and community resources further in the following chapters.

- Social work practitioners should include all family members in service delivery either directly or by referring family members to other professionals or peers. This supports the family system, which also impacts the child's mental health.
- Social work advocacy has to work on expanding family services as well as the expansion of environmental supports such as workplace flexibility, paid leave, and other economic support programs to reduce family stressors.

Part 7: Application for Social Work Education

Social work education can play a critical role in preparing future practitioners to adequately support families caring for a child with a mental health disability. For example, courses focused on mental health assessment and interventions could include one session on how a child's mental health diagnosis might affect the whole family including parents as well as siblings or other relatives. Courses on family interventions could add information about the importance of economic security for family resilience. This can go beyond a discussion of welfare programs and include information about issues of work-life fit, workplace flexibility, and workplace policies such as paid family and medical leave or family responsibility workplace discrimination.

Case Scenario

Julia (mother, 42), Robert (father, 47), Maria (daughter, 12), and Ben (son, 10). Hunter just moved to a new state, because Robert was offered a better-paying position at a non-profit agency. Julia is currently looking for a new position as an accountant. Money is tighter right now, since Julia is not working. Maria and Ben are both enrolled in public schools, Maria in a large middle school and Ben in a small elementary school. Maria has recently been diagnosed with depression and an eating disorder, which upended the family's routines. Maria participates in an out-patient half-day treatment program. Julia is driving Maria to the clinic at 8 am in the morning and picks her up at 1 pm. Robert is helping Ben in the mornings and makes sure he gets on the school bus before heading to work. Maria is not going to school right now and has to be supervised. Maria and Julia spend the afternoon together until they pick up Ben from school. Robert often comes home late from work, since he is still learning his new job. Luckily, Robert's job comes with good health insurance, and the out-of-pocket payments for Maria's current treatment are manageable. The family doesn't have friends yet, since they just moved to the new town. Julia and Robert left behind their parents and siblings. While they don't have any family members in the area, they all feel very connected to each other. Ben has been acting out at home and at school. His school has called his parents for a meeting, since Ben hit another schoolmate in a fight over the monkey bars. You are a social worker in Maria's clinic, and you work with the family members of the children receiving treatment.

ACTIVITY 1: WORKING WITH FAMILY HUNTER

Competency 2: Advance Human Rights and Social, Racial, Economic, and Environmental Justice

Competency 3: Engage Anti-Racism, Diversity, Equity, and Inclusion (ADEI) in Practice

Competency 6: Engage with Individuals, Families, Groups, Organizations, and Communities
Competency 7: Assess Individuals, Families, Groups, Organizations, and Communities
Competency 8: Intervene with Individuals, Families, Groups, Organizations, and Communities

First, role play your first meeting with family Hunter using the above scenario as a starting point.

Second, conduct a bio-psycho-social-spiritual assessment including both areas of struggle and areas of strength for all individual members and for the family as a whole.

Third, develop an intervention plan for the family based on your assessment.

- What referrals would you suggest?
- Who else would you like to get involved?
- Include interventions that can increase individual and family coping, social connectedness, and economic security.

Fourth, discuss the following alternatives:

- How would the scenario change if the family did not have good health insurance and there was no treatment spot available?
- How would the scenario change if the family was embedded in a supportive community?
- How would the scenario change if both parents worked and could not take time off to manage Maria's treatment?

ACTIVITY 2: CONNECTING POLICY AND FAMILY RESILIENCE

Competency 2: Advance Human Rights and Social, Racial, Economic, and Environmental Justice
Competency 3: Engage Anti-Racism, Diversity, Equity, and Inclusion (ADEI) in Practice
Competency 5: Engage in Policy Practice

Research current policies related to health insurance and paid leave. Apply the social-ecological framework of resilience introduced in this chapter and discuss the following questions:

- How can these policies strengthen family resilience?
- How might these policies add stressors negatively affecting family adaptation?
- What changes are necessary to better support family resilience?

Resource List

Caregiver strain scale available at the School of Nursing & Health Studies Center of Excellence for Health Disparities Research at the University of Miami https://elcentro.sonhs.miami.edu/research/measures-library/cgsq/index.html

Key processes in family resilience from Walsh, F. (2006). *Strengthening family resilience.* Guilford Press, New York, NY. including:

Belief systems

- Making meaning of adversity
- Positive outlook
- Transcendence and spirituality

Organizational patterns

- Flexibility
- Connectedness
- Social and economic resources

Communication processes

- Clarity
- Open and emotional expression
- Collaborative problem solving

Family-Run Executive Director Leadership Association: https://www.fredla.org/
National Alliance on Mental Illness: https://www.nami.org/
National Federation of Families: https://www.ffcmh.org/
Family support recommendations: British Psychological Society Division (2021). Family interventions in psychosis. Guidelines for psychologists and practitioners supporting families and social networks. https://explore.bps.org.uk/binary/bpsworks/8d5e93f37ef93aa0/6f9b1f52231c12bfd96fd69f80b38e60af29eedac01780db9a8c909e2a85ee4a/rep151_2021.pdf

References

Abbott, M., Bernard, P., & Forge, J. (2013). Communicating a diagnosis of Autism Spectrum Disorder – A qualitative study of parents' experiences. *Clinical Child Psychology and Psychiatry, 18*(3), 370–382. https://doi.org/10.1177/1359104512455813

Abrams, S. M. (2009). The well sibling: Challenges and possibilities. *American Journal of Psychotherapy, 63*(4), 305–317. https://doi.org/10.1176/appi.psychotherapy.2009.63.4.305.

Barnable, A., Gaudine, A., Bennett, L., & Maedus, R. (2006). Having a sibling with schizophrenia: A phenomenological study. *Research and Theory of Nursing Practice: An International Journal, 20*(3), 247–264. https://doi.org/10.1891/rtnp.20.3.247.

Boss, P. (1999). *Ambiguous loss: Learning to live with unresolved grief* (1st ed.). Harvard University Press. https://doi.org/10.4159/9780674028586

Bourke-Taylor, H., Pallant, J. F., Law, M., Howie, L. (2012). Predicting mental health among mothers of school-aged children with developmental disabilities: The relative contribution of child, maternal and environmental factors. *Research Developmental Disability, 33*(6), 1732–1740. https://doi.org/10.1016/j.ridd.2012.04.011.

Brannan, A. M., Brennan, E. M., Sellmaier, C., & Rosenzweig, J. M. (2018). Employed parents of children receiving mental health services: Caregiver strain and work-life integration. *Families in Society, 99*(1), 29–44. https://doi.org/10.1177/1044389418756375

Brannan, A. M., Heflinger, C. A., & Bickman, L. (1997). The caregiver strain questionnaire: Measuring the impact on the family of living with a child with serious emotional disturbance. *Journal of Emotional and Behavioral Disorders, 5*, 212–222. https://doi.org/10.1177/106342669700500404

Brown, M., Whiting, J., Kahumoku-Fessler, E., Witting, A. B. & Jensen, J. (2020). A dyadic model of stress, coping, and marital satisfaction among parents of children with autism. *Family Relations, 69*, 138–150. https://doi.org/10.1111/fare.12375

Churchill, S. S., Villareale, N. L., Monaghan, T. A., Sharp, V. L., & Kieckhefer, G. M. (2010). Parents of children with special health care needs who have better coping skills have fewer depressive symptoms. *Maternal Child and Health Journal, 14*, 47–57. https://doi.org/10.1007/s10995-008-0435-0

Coltrane, S., Miller, E. C., DeHaan, T., & Stewart, L. (2013). Fathers and the flexibility stigma. *Journal of Social Issues, 69*(2), 279–302. https://doi.org/10.1111/josi.12015

Friesen, B. J. (1989). *Survey of parents whose children have serious emotional disorders: Report of a National Study*. Research and Training Center on Family Support and Children's Mental Health, Portland State University.

Grzywacz, J. G., & Marks, N. F. (2000). Reconceptualizing the work-family interface: An ecological perspective on the correlates of positive and negative spillover between work and family. *Journal of Occupational Health Psychology, 5*, 111–126. https://doi.org/10.1037/1076-8998.5.1.111

Ha, J. H., Hong, J., Seltzer, M. M., & Greenberg, J. S. (2008). Age and gender differences in the well-being of midlife and aging parents with children with mental health or developmental problems: Report of a national study. *Journal of Health and Social Behavior*, 49, 301–316. https://doi.org/10.1177/002214650804900305

Harden, J. (2005). Parenting a young person with mental health problems: Temporal disruption and reconstruction. *Sociology of Health & Illness, 27*(3), 351–371. https://doi.org/10.1111/j.1467-9566.2005.00446.x

Hartley, S. L., Papp, L. M., & Bolt, D. (2018). Spillover of marital interactions and parenting stress in families of children with autism spectrum disorder. *Journal of Clinical Child & Adolescent Psychology, 47*(S1), S88–S99. https://doi.org/10.1080/15374416.2016.1152552

Jin, Y., & Mazrekaj, D. (2025). A comparison of health and well-being between same-sex and different-sex parents: A systematic review and recommendations for future research. *Genus, 81*(1), Article 25. https://doi.org/10.1186/s41118-025-00266-z

Kendall, J., & Shelton, K. (2003). A typology of family management styles in families with children with ADHD. *Journal of Family Nursing, 9*(3), 257–280. https://doi.org/10.1177/1074840703255446

Kvist, A. P., Nielsen, H. S., & Simonsen, M. (2013). The importance of children's ADHD for parents' relationship stability and labor supply. *Social Science and Medicine, 80*, 30–38. https://doi.org/10.1016/j.socscimed.2013.04.001.

Levante, A., Martis, C., Del Prete, C. M., Martino, P., Primiceri, P., & Lecciso, F. (2024). Siblings of persons with disabilities: A systematic integrative review of the empirical literature. *Clinical Child and Family Psychology Review, 28*(2), 209–253. https://doi.org/10.1007/s10567-024-00502-6

Lewis, S., Kagan, C., Heaton, P., & Cranshaw, M. (1999). Economic and psychological benefits from employment: The experiences and perspectives of mothers of disabled children. *Disability & Society, 14*(4), 561–575. https://doi.org/10.1080/09687599926127

Lively, S., Friedrich, R. M., & Buckwalter, K. C. (1995). Sibling perception of schizophrenia: Impact on relationships, roles, and health. *Issues in Mental Health Nursing*, *16*(3), 225–238. https://doi.org/10.3109/01612849509006937

McCabe, K. M., Yeh, M., Lau, A., Garland, A., & Hough, R. (2003). Racial/ethnic differences in caregiver strain and perceived social support among parents of youth with emotional and behavioral problems. *Mental Health Services Research*, *5*(3), 137–147. https://doi.org/10.1023/A:1024439317884

McCann, T. V., Lubman, D. I., & Clark, E. (2011). First-time primary caregivers' experience of caring for young adults with first-episode psychosis. *Schizophrenia Bulletin*, *37*(2), 381–388. https://doi.org/10.1093/schbul/sbp085

McConnell, D., Savage, A., & Breitkreuz, R. (2014). Resilience in families raising children with disabilities and behavior problems. *Research in Developmental Disabilities*, *35*, 833–848. https://doi.org/10.1016/j.ridd.2014.01.015

Minnotte, K. L., Minnotte, M. C., & Bonstrom, J. (2015). Work–family conflicts and marital satisfaction among US workers: Does stress amplification matter? *Journal of Family and Economic Issues*, *36*(1), 21–33. https://doi.org/10.1007/s10834-014-9420-5

O'Brien, M. (2007). Ambiguous loss in families of children with Autism Spectrum Disorders. *Family Relations*, *56*, 135–146. https://doi-org.offcampus.lib.washington.edu/10.1111/j.1741-3729.2007.00447.x

Patterson, J. M. (2002). Integrating family resilience and family stress theory. *Journal of Marriage and Family*, *64*, 349–360. https://doi.org/10.1111/j.1741-3737.2002.00349.x

Quittner, A. L, Espelage, D. L, & Opipari, L. C. (1998). Role strain in couples with and without a child with a chronic illness: Associations with marital satisfaction, intimacy, and daily mood. *Health Psychology*, *17*(2), 112–124. https://doi.org/10.1037/0278-6133.17.2.112

Riebschleger, J. L. (1991). Families of chronically mentally ill people: Siblings speak to social workers. *Health and Social Work*, *16*(2), 94–103. https://doi.org/10.1093/hsw/16.2.94.

Sellmaier, C. (2019). Integrating work and family responsibilities: Experiences of fathers of children with special health care needs. *Journal of Child and Family Studies*, *28*(11), 3022–3036. https://doi.org/10.1007/s10826-019-01478-6

Sellmaier, C. (2021). Physical and mental health of mothers and fathers caring for children with special health care needs: The influence of community resources. *Journal of Family Issues*, *43*(11), 2815–2840. https://doi.org/10.1177/0192513X211035580

Sellmaier, C., & Buckingham, S. (2022). "I think sometimes that dads are kind of forgotten (…) so it's nice that we also get a voice.": Work-life experiences of employed U.S. fathers caring for a child with special health care needs. *Community, Work, & Family*, *25*(5), 661–676. https://doi.org/10.1080/13668803.2021.1911935

Sellmaier, C., Stewart, L. M., & Brennan, E. M. (2020). Workforce engagement of parents of children and youth with mental health difficulties: The impact of community services and supports. *Community Work & Family*, *23*(5), 534–555. https://doi.org/10.1080/13668803.2020.1820954

Stewart, L., Sellmaier, C., Henderson-Posther, M., Brennan, E. M., & Lukefahr, J. (2024). Navigating family responsibility discrimination: Parenting a child with a mental health disability. In P. Neff Claster, & S. L. Blair: (Eds.), *Contemporary perspectives in family research* (p. 27). Emerald Publishing.

Stewart, L. M., Sellmaier, C., Brannan, A. M., & Brennan, E. M. (2023). Family demands and workplace supports of employed parents of children with typical and exceptional care responsibilities and their effects on conflict and stress. *Journal of Child and Family Studies*, *32*(4), 1048–1064. https://doi.org/10.1007/s10826-022-02363-5

Ungar, M. (2011). The social ecology of resilience: Addressing contextual and cultural ambiguity of a nascent construct. *American Journal of Orthopsychiatry*, *81*, 1–17. https://doi.org/10.1111/j.1939-0025.2010.01067.x

Van Der Sanden, R. L. M., Bos, A. E. R., Stutterheim, S. E., Pryor, J. B., & Kok, G. (2015). Stigma by association among family members of people with a mental illness: A qualitative analysis. *Journal of Community & Applied Social Psychology*, *25*(5), 400–417. https://doi.org/10.1002/casp.2221

Walsh, F. (2003). Family resilience: A framework for family practice. *Family Process*, *42*(1), 1–18. https://doi.org/10.1111/j.1545-5300.2003.00001.x

Walsh, F. (2006). *Strengthening family resilience*. Guilford Press.

5

THE WORK–FAMILY DILEMMA

The challenges parents face when raising a child with a mental health disability are not limited to just understanding their child's mental health needs or obtaining a diagnosis. Equally important is the ongoing work of integrating caregiving responsibilities with paid employment while navigating complex systems of care. Parents must coordinate services across health care, education, and community settings in ways that directly shape their capacity to remain employed, meet workplace expectations, and sustain family functioning. This coordination requires sustained advocacy, administrative labor, and emotional effort, often in contexts that are under-resourced, poorly coordinated, and difficult to access (Brannan et al., 2018; Sellmaier & Buckingham, 2022).

This chapter draws on the concept of work–family integration to examine how caregiving and employment are deeply interconnected in parents' everyday lives (Lewis, 2003; Lewis et al., 2007). For parents of children with mental health disabilities, care demands are often unpredictable, episodic, and long term, complicating efforts to align work schedules, job expectations, and family needs. Role theory helps explain how these competing demands generate role strain when workplace expectations conflict with caregiving responsibilities or when parents are required to perform multiple roles simultaneously without adequate support (Pleck, 1977). These challenges are further intensified by stigmatizing attitudes toward behaviors associated with mental illness, which can constrain access to workplace flexibility and undermine accommodation efforts (Corrigan & Miller, 2004; Goffman, 1963; Rosenzweig & Huffstutter, 2004). Framing caregiving through a work–family integration lens highlights how employment outcomes are shaped not only by individual coping strategies, but by organizational norms, institutional supports, and social responses to mental health and disability caregiving.

DOI: 10.4324/9781003532668-5

The misalignment between caregiving demands and workplace expectations is not abstract. Parents described situations in which the unpredictable and intensive nature of their child's mental health needs was interpreted through rigid workplace norms that left little room for accommodation.

As one parent explained when reflecting on an interaction with a supervisor:

> She told me that she wouldn't be a good supervisor if she didn't give me a heads up that this is what she was seeing. She said I was having trouble with my competing priorities and that I had to get it together somehow.
>
> *(Stewart & Charles, 2021)*

This experience is not unique. It illustrates what is at the heart of exceptional caregiving, responsibilities shaped by crises, that are reoccurring and garner uncertainty that is reframed as an individual's shortcoming rather than as evidence of structural incompatibility. Parents are not recognized as managing competing systems of responsibility, but as failing to meet implicit norms of the ideal worker (Williams, 2000). This misfit intensifies role strain and shapes subsequent decisions about disclosure, flexibility use, and continued attachment to the labor force.

In this chapter, work–family dilemmas faced by parents of children with mental health disabilities are examined by centering caregiving as a form of labor embedded within broader social, organizational, and policy contexts. We situate work–family integration within established work–family theory, examine the time bind created by *crisis-oriented care*, analyze the workplace flexibility dilemma and threats to job security, and explore how the disclosure and stigma processes shape parents' employment decisions. We then consider the cumulative financial strain associated with mental health-related caregiving and conclude by examining the conditional circumstances under which work can function as a stabilizing and protective force. Together, these analyses highlight how employment outcomes for parents of children with mental health disabilities are shaped not only by caregiving intensity, but by the degree to which they are able to navigate workplaces and systems of care that are not structured to accommodate the realities of mental health disability across the life course. This chapter draws in part on qualitative interviews with employed parents of children with mental health disabilities conducted as part of a multi-study research program examining work, caregiving, and disclosure decision-making.

Part 1: Understanding Work–Family Integration

The concept of work–family integration builds on decades of scholarship examining how individuals navigate their roles as workers and caregivers. Early work–family research focused heavily on work–family balance, the idea that well-being depends on maintaining equilibrium between competing demands at home and at work (Greenhaus & Allen, 2011). Balance-oriented frameworks tend to assume caregiving demands that are predictable, time-limited, and socially recognized, and they place primary responsibility on individuals to manage competing roles through personal strategies and employer-provided flexibility (Lewis et al., 2007; Voydanoff, 2007). While useful for understanding some caregiving contexts, these assumptions poorly reflect the realities of parents raising children with mental health disabilities.

In response to these limitations, work–family and disability scholars increasingly emphasized concepts such as work–family fit and integration, which foreground alignment between caregiving demands and employment contexts rather than individual equilibrium. Rosenzweig et al. (2002) were among the first to apply the notion of work-family fit to parents of children with emotional and behavioral disorders, arguing that parents seek compatibility between family needs and workplace structures rather than balance per se. From this perspective, work–family fit reflects how well job demands, organizational culture, workplace supports, and available community resources correspond to the realities of disability-related caregiving (Rosenzweig et al., 2008).

This work was later extended using national data from the National Study of the Changing Workforce, developed by Galinsky and colleagues to capture how job conditions, organizational culture, and caregiving demands interact to shape workers' well-being and labor force attachment in the United States (Galinsky et al., 2011). Using data from the 2004 and 2016 waves, Stewart (2009, 2013) and Stewart et al. (2022*a*) found that employed parents providing exceptional care reported significantly higher levels of work–family conflict, family–work conflict, and stress than parents providing typical care. These differences persisted after accounting for personal and family characteristics, indicating that misfit is not explained by individual capacity or family structure alone, but by how workplaces are organized to respond, or fail to respond, to complex and unpredictable care demands. Role theory helps illuminate how this misfit is experienced in everyday work contexts. Role strain emerges when individuals occupy multiple roles governed by incompatible expectations and limited flexibility (Pleck, 1977). For parents managing mental health-related caregiving, role strain is intensified by the need to respond to crises that cannot be scheduled, delegated, or postponed (Rosenzweig et al., 2002). Parents described workplace interactions in which this incompatibility was framed not as a structural issue but as a personal failing.

As one parent explained:

> There are some people in my department that I don't feel comfortable sharing really personal stuff with, because I'm not convinced that they won't use it against me or share it with other people I don't want to know.

This account reflects work–family misfit at the level of organizational interpretation, where caregiving responsibilities are perceived as potential liabilities rather than legitimate constraints. In such contexts, parents must manage not only competing role demands but also ongoing threats to professional credibility, shaping how, when, and whether they seek support at work. Rosenzweig et al. (2011) described this dynamic as *feeding the rumor mill.*

Stigmatizing attitudes toward mental illness further compound work–family misfit by shaping how caregiving demands are evaluated in workplace settings. Mental health-related caregiving is often less visible and less socially sanctioned than other forms of care, increasing the likelihood that parents will be judged as unreliable or insufficiently committed (Goffman, 1963; Stewart et al., 2025). Parents in our interviews described how such judgments eroded their credibility at work. This diminished legitimacy reflects the operation of ideal worker norms, which assume employees are unencumbered by caregiving and able to prioritize work consistently (Williams, 2000). When parents of children with mental health disabilities fall short of these expectations due to caregiving demands, misfit is individualized and moralized rather than recognized as a structural incompatibility (Rosenzweig & Huffstutter, 2004; Stewart et al., 2025).

Ecological perspectives on work–family integration emphasize that alignment is shaped not only within workplaces but across work, family, and community systems (Voydanoff, 2007). Drawing on this framework, Sellmaier et al. (2020) analyzed a national child health dataset and found that access to coordinated community services plays a critical role in moderating work–family misfit. When mental health services, school supports, and community-based resources are fragmented or unavailable, parents experience heightened employment precarity, as job stability becomes contingent on the timing and intensity of care crises. In these contexts, misfit emerges simultaneously across systems, reinforcing strain and constraining parents' employment options. We will further discuss the role of community resources in Chapter 6.

Part 2: The Time Bind and the Crisis-Oriented Nature of Care

Parenting a child with a mental health disability produces a distinctive form of what Hochschild (1997) described as the *time bind*, a compression of time created by the collision of employment demands and caregiving responsibilities. For parents in this context, time strain is not simply a matter of having too much to do, but of managing care demands that are unpredictable, episodic, and crisis-driven within systems that are fragmented and often broken. This form of caregiving rarely conforms to routines or schedules and instead requires parents to remain in a state of constant readiness, reorganizing work and family life around sudden escalations and interruptions reflecting the etiology of the child's mental health and developmental trajectory. Care responsibilities include crisis response, advocacy within schools, and coordination with health and mental health providers, expanding the scope of caregiving well beyond typical parenting and embedding crisis management into daily life. The care is further marginalized by fewer social supports as the emotional and behavioral needs of the child require that caregivers understand how to maintain child and caregiver safety as well as manage the child's physical and emotional behaviors.

Mental health-related caregiving is distinguished not only by its intensity but by its volatility. Children's needs may escalate suddenly, requiring immediate parental attention due to behavioral crises, school exclusions, psychiatric hospitalization, or abrupt service disruptions. These events do not merely interrupt daily routines but reorganize parents' work lives around constant contingency.

As one parent described:

> If the school calls, you can't just not pick up the phone. Usually, if it's the school, it's something like, 'Hey, I need you to call me right now.' So, you know, it's that kind of stuff…her mental health, some days is worse than others, for sure.

This account illustrates how work is performed under conditions of *constant readiness* rather than *temporal separation or segmentation*, a defining feature of crisis-driven caregiving. Parents must anticipate potential disruptions and remain available to respond, even when physically present at work. These temporal disruptions are compounded by the fragmented nature of community-based mental health services. When school-based supports, wraparound services, respite care, or in-home therapy are limited or poorly coordinated, parents are forced to absorb additional care labor during the workday (Sellmaier et al., 2020). Employment stability becomes contingent on whether and when crises occur, producing a form of employment precarity tied directly to care contingencies (Stewart et al., 2022b).

The cumulative result is a deepening of the time bind. Parents' caregiving responsibilities expand in scope and unpredictability, while their paid work becomes increasingly vulnerable to disruption. Empirical research consistently shows that parents of children with emotional and behavioral disorders experience higher rates of absenteeism, reduced work hours, and employment loss than parents in other caregiving contexts (Brennan et al., 2016; Rosenzweig et al., 2008). Importantly, these outcomes reflect structural incompatibilities between crisis-driven care and rigid work expectations rather than diminished work commitment.

The emotional labor required to manage this constant state of contingency further intensifies time strain. Parents must monitor their child's well-being, anticipate crises, and manage uncertainty while attempting to maintain professional credibility at work. This vigilance contributes to fatigue, burnout, and cumulative stress, particularly in workplaces that lack flexibility or interpret interruptions as evidence of unreliability (Sellmaier, 2019). Access to coordinated and family-centered community supports can moderate the effects of the time bind. Parents who can draw on integrated systems of care report fewer work disruptions and improved well-being (Stewart et al., 2022a). However, such supports remain unevenly distributed and are often inaccessible to families facing additional structural barriers related to socioeconomic status, geography, or race. As a result, the time bind operates as an inequitable burden, reinforcing disparities in both caregiving and employment outcomes.

The time bind experienced by parents of children with mental health disabilities is shaped not only by the quantity of caregiving required, but by its crisis-driven and temporally disorganizing nature. It reflects the misalignment between caregiving realities and workplace expectations, compounded by fragmented service systems that externalize crisis management onto families. Recognizing this form of *time strain* is essential for understanding why flexibility, disclosure, and employment stability are so tightly bound for parents navigating mental health–related caregiving.

Part 3: The Workplace Flexibility Dilemma and Employment Precarity

For parents of children with mental health disabilities, workplace flexibility is not a discretionary benefit or a work–life preference. It is a condition for continued employment. The crisis-driven *time bind* described in Part 2 makes flexibility essential for responding to school calls, emergency appointments, hospitalization, and periods of heightened supervision needs. Yet access to flexibility is uneven, frequently informal, and often contingent on managerial discretion. As a result, the parents who most need flexibility are often those least protected when using it.

Workplace flexibility scholars have emphasized that flexibility is not inherently supportive and can, under certain conditions, reproduce inequality and risk (Kossek et al., 2021). Flexible arrangements are most protective when they are formalized, equitably available, and embedded within supportive organizational cultures. When flexibility is informal, negotiated individually, or unevenly monitored, it can become a source of employment precarity rather than accommodation. Parents' accounts illustrate how flexibility often functions as a fragile and revocable resource. Flexibility arrangements were described as highly person-dependent, requiring repeated renegotiation as supervisors changed or organizational priorities shifted.

One parent explained:

> I've honestly had four different bosses since this whole situation started, and that's been the hardest thing, because I feel like a broken record… I have to keep trying to let them know what's going on, just because I don't want my merit decreased or anything because of what's happened.

This account highlights how flexibility that is not institutionalized must be continually re-earned. Each new supervisory relationship resets the terms of accommodation, exposing parents to renewed scrutiny and performance risk. In these contexts, flexibility operates as a conditional privilege rather than a stable employment support.

Even when flexibility is granted, parents remain acutely aware of its reputational costs. Flexibility use was often accompanied by fear of being perceived as less committed or less reliable, a dynamic consistent with research on *flexibility stigma* (Kossek et al., 2021). For parents managing mental health–related caregiving, this stigma is intensified by the unpredictability of care demands, the frequency of interruptions and the *courtesy stigma* assigned because of the child's mental health etiology (Corrigan & Miller, 2004; Stewart et al., 2025).

When flexibility proves insufficient or unsafe to use, parents may reduce hours, accept downgraded roles, or exit employment altogether. These decisions were rarely framed as preferences. Instead, parents described leaving work or scaling back after being unable to navigate opaque or poorly communicated protections, reflecting structural failure rather than individual choice (Brown & Clark, 2017; Rosenzweig et al., 2002).

Even when parents remained employed, flexibility sometimes functioned as a *one-way accommodation*. Temporary reductions in hours or responsibilities made during periods of crisis were later normalized, resulting in permanent reductions in pay, benefits, or advancement opportunities. One parent described this dynamic succinctly:

> I went down to 30 hours, and I was still able to do the job. Now he doesn't want to bring me back up to 40 hours because he's seen I can do it. He's able to pay me less, I get fewer benefits, and that's just kind of the price of the flexible arrangement.

This account illustrates how flexibility can operate as a ratchet, capturing productivity while externalizing long-term risk onto workers. These findings underscore the notion that workplace flexibility operates at the intersection of *time*, *stigma*, and *power*. When flexibility is individualized and unsafe to use, it becomes a mechanism through which work–family fit is managed privately rather than addressed structurally. This dynamic sets the stage for parents' subsequent disclosure decisions, which are shaped less by openness than by ongoing risk calculation.

Part 4: Disclosure under Courtesy Stigma and Flexible Precarity

For parents of children with mental health disabilities, disclosure is not a discrete event or a purely communicative choice. It is an ongoing process of risk management shaped by courtesy stigma, employment precarity, and moralized expectations of parenting (Rosenzweig et al., 2011; Stewart & Charles, 2021). Unlike disclosure involving one's own health condition or episodic caregiving for an aging parent, disclosure in this context exposes parents to judgments about both worker reliability and parental competence.

BOX 5.1 CASE SNAPSHOT: DISCLOSURE DURING CRISIS

Calvin is a facilities manager at a large public university. He is the parent of a 16-year-old daughter, Riley, who has bipolar disorder. Riley's condition is episodic. For long stretches, she attends school regularly and manages well with outpatient support. During periods of escalation, however, Riley experiences severe mood instability, sleep disruption, and suicidal ideation that requires constant supervision and, at times, hospitalization.

Calvin has intentionally avoided disclosing Riley's diagnosis at work. His position is operational and visibility-dependent, and he supervises a team responsible for campus safety and maintenance. Although his job includes some flexibility, it also involves being on call for emergencies. Calvin has previously relied on accrued leave, informal shift swaps, and vague references to "family issues" to manage Riley's needs.

The crisis

One evening, Riley experiences a rapid escalation and is taken to the emergency department for psychiatric evaluation. Calvin remains with her overnight. The following morning, he is scheduled to oversee a critical facilities inspection tied to regulatory compliance. For the first time, concealment is no longer viable. Calvin realizes that he cannot meet work obligations without immediate, explicit communication.

Step 1: Crisis overrides planning

In contrast to anticipatory decision-making, Calvin's disclosure is forced by immediacy. There is no opportunity to test responses gradually or limit information flow. His priority shifts from managing stigma to ensuring safety and continuity of care.

Factors in play:

Crisis status, urgency, collapse of concealment

Step 2: Strategic disclosure to multiple actors

Calvin contacts his supervisor and human resources the same morning. He discloses that his daughter is experiencing a psychiatric emergency and requires hospitalization, and that he will need immediate leave. He does not provide diagnostic labels initially, but the severity of the situation is clear.

Disclosure strategies in play:

Full disclosure driven by necessity

Step 3: Organizational response and risk exposure

The response is procedurally supportive. Human resources provides information about medical leave and job protection. However, Calvin also experiences heightened scrutiny. He is asked to provide documentation quickly, clarify timelines, and delegate responsibilities indefinitely. While his job is protected in the short term, he becomes aware that leadership is questioning his ability to manage an on-call role long term.

Calvin begins to worry not about job loss, but about reassignment, loss of supervisory authority, or future exclusion from leadership roles.

Step 4: After the crisis, new calculations

When Riley stabilizes and returns home, Calvin does not "return to baseline." Disclosure has permanently altered how his availability is perceived. He now weighs future decisions differently, including whether to request a modified role, pursue advancement, or seek employment with more predictable demands.

Disclosure outcome illustrated:

Disclosure outcomes feed forward into future risk assessments

Traditional workplace disclosure scholarship emphasizes authenticity, boundary management, and access to accommodation (Clair et al., 2005; Ragins, 2008). In contrast, disclosure by parents of children with mental health disabilities is shaped by *courtesy stigma*, whereby negative evaluations attached to a child's condition extend to the parent (Corrigan & Miller, 2004; Goffman, 1963). Behavioral and emotional challenges associated with children's mental health are frequently interpreted as failures of parenting rather than manifestations of disability, producing a qualitatively different disclosure terrain (Rosenzweig et al., 2011; Stewart et al., 2018, 2025).

This distinction is well documented in the work of Rosenzweig and colleagues. Early qualitative studies showed that parents framed disclosure decisions around fears of being judged as irresponsible, unreliable, or incapable of managing family life (Rosenzweig et al., 2002). Subsequent research demonstrated that disclosure often triggered scrutiny not only of parents' work performance, but of their values and moral standing as parents, with discipline enacted through attendance expectations, time-based metrics, and informal supervisory evaluations that failed to account for crisis-driven care (Rosenzweig et al., 2008, 2011).

More recent work situates these dynamics within contemporary flexibility regimes. Parents providing exceptional care experience higher levels of work–family conflict and stress than parents providing typical care, even when workplace supports are nominally available (Stewart et al., 2022a). Organizational support appears protective only when flexibility is safe to use and not accompanied by stigma or surveillance (Kossek et al., 2021). As a result, disclosure decisions cannot be separated from how flexibility is structured, monitored, and evaluated.

Parents' accounts illustrate how disclosure is carefully calibrated rather than all-or-nothing. Disclosure is often partial, strategic, and timed to prevent misinterpretation while limiting vulnerability (Rosenzweig et al., 2011).

As one parent explained:

> I definitely thought about and planned out in advance what I was going to say and thought about the timing of the ask…the whole strategy around it.

Partial disclosure allowed parents to legitimize flexibility use without fully reclassifying themselves as problematic workers or parents. However, it also required ongoing vigilance and impression management, particularly as crises recurred or accommodations extended over time (Rosenzweig et al., 2011).

Affective considerations further shaped disclosure decisions. Parents described embarrassment, fear of being judged, and concern about being viewed as replaceable, reflecting deeply embedded ideal worker norms that assume employees should manage family issues privately and without disrupting work (Stewart et al., 2025; Williams, 2000). These fears were not hypothetical. Parents who disclosed and used flexibility during crises sometimes experienced longer-term career penalties, including stalled advancement or permanent downgrading of roles (Stewart & Charles, 2021).

Evidence from studies examining workplace disclosure as a strategy suggests that disclosure for parents of children with mental health disabilities operates as a distinct workplace context. It is shaped by courtesy stigma, moralized expectations of parenting, and crisis driven and cyclical care needs that can transform short-term accommodations into long-term disadvantage. Parents are not simply deciding whether to disclose. They are continually assessing how much risk they can afford to take to sustain both caregiving and employment under conditions where the costs of miscalculation are cumulative and difficult to reverse. Understanding disclosure through this lens clarifies why parents engage in anticipatory planning, partial disclosure, and ongoing impression management. These strategies are not signs of avoidance or lack of authenticity, but rational responses to structural conditions that render full transparency risky. In this context, disclosure functions less as a pathway to accommodation than as a site where work–family fit, stigma, and employment precarity converge.

Part 5: The Financial Strain Associated with Caring for a Child with a Mental Health Disability

The financial strain experienced by parents raising children with mental health disabilities is not solely the result of direct care costs. Rather, it reflects a cumulative process through which caregiving demands interact with labor market structures, workplace practices, and policy gaps to produce economic vulnerability over time. As the preceding sections demonstrated, employment precarity, flexibility penalties, and constrained disclosure decisions shape parents' work trajectories. These dynamics, in turn, translate directly into financial strain.

Early evidence of these economic penalties can be found in Warfield's research on parents caring for children with emotional and behavioral disorders. Warfield (2005) documented reduced labor force participation, elevated role strain, and heightened employment disruption among parents whose children required intensive mental health support. Importantly, these penalties emerged not simply from time demands but from the unpredictability and emotional intensity of care, characteristics that distinguish mental health caregiving from other disability contexts.

Subsequent research has demonstrated that these early employment disruptions translate into longer-term economic vulnerability. Parish and colleagues showed that parents of children with disabilities experience reduced labor force participation, lower earnings, and diminished access to employer-sponsored benefits across the life course (Parish & Cloud, 2006; Parish et al., 2004). These penalties persist even among parents who remain employed, underscoring that labor force attachment alone does not guarantee economic security when caregiving demands are chronic and crisis driven.

DeRigne's work further clarifies how caregiving-related employment disruption produces material hardship. Parents of children with special health care needs face elevated risks of income instability, benefit loss, and unmet basic needs when caregiving interferes with work continuity (DeRigne, 2012; DeRigne & Porterfield, 2017). Reductions in hours, transitions to part-time work, or exits from employment typically occur in response to care crises rather than preference, reinforcing the argument that financial strain is structurally produced rather than individually chosen.

Research by Porterfield and colleagues highlights how these employment disruptions interact with gaps in workplace benefits and public supports. Families are often forced to rely on a patchwork of unpaid leave, employer-based benefits, and out-of-pocket spending, particularly when children's mental health needs fall outside narrowly defined eligibility criteria for public assistance (Porterfield & DeRigne, 2011; DeRigne & Porterfield, 2017). For parents of children with mental health disabilities, whose care needs are episodic and poorly aligned with categorical service systems, this misalignment is especially pronounced.

Work–family scholarship situates these financial penalties within broader organizational and policy contexts. Disability, work and family scholars argue that institutional arrangements that privatize care responsibility and assume uninterrupted labor force attachment shift economic risk onto families when caregiving needs intensify (Lewis et al., 2007). In such contexts, flexible work arrangements, when poorly protected, can exacerbate economic insecurity by normalizing reduced hours, stalled careers, and long-term earnings penalties rather than preventing them.

The qualitative data used in this chapter reinforce these patterns. Parents described making financially consequential employment decisions, including reducing hours, accepting lower pay, or remaining in downgraded positions to preserve flexibility and health insurance. These decisions were rarely framed as voluntary trade-offs. Instead, they were understood as necessary adaptations to systems that offered limited support for crisis-driven care, illustrating how financial penalties become normalized within caregiving contexts. Financial strain also feeds back into parents' disclosure and employment decisions. Concerns about income loss, benefit eligibility, and long-term security shape how much flexibility parents can afford to use and how much information they are willing to disclose at work (DeRigne & Porterfield, 2017; Stewart et al., 2022a). Parents with fewer financial buffers are more likely to conceal caregiving needs or remain in precarious employment arrangements to minimize risk, reinforcing work–family misfit over time.

Taken together, the evidence shows that financial strain among parents of children with mental health disabilities reflects a structural pattern of cumulative disadvantage produced at the intersection of caregiving demands, workplace practices, and policy gaps. Families are not simply managing higher costs but navigating labor market conditions that systematically devalue caregiving and externalize economic risk. Understanding financial strain through this lens is essential for developing workplace, policy, and social service interventions that move beyond short-term accommodations toward long-term economic security.

Part 6: The Conditional and Protective Role of Work

Although much of the literature emphasizes financial strain and employment disruption, scholars caution against framing paid work solely as a source of burden for parents raising children with mental health disabilities. Research spanning more than two decades demonstrates that employment can function as a protective, stabilizing, and identity-affirming resource, but only under specific conditions. The benefits of work are conditional rather than automatic, shaped by the degree to which employment structures align with the realities of crisis-driven caregiving.

Across work–family, disability, and caregiving scholarship, four interrelated domains capture the circumstances under which work can play a positive role: economic stability, psychological well-being and identity, social connection, and structure and respite from caregiving intensity.

Economic Stability and Material Security

Continued attachment to the labor force provides critical economic resources that support family stability and access to care. In the United States, employment remains the primary pathway to income, health insurance, and employment-based benefits essential for mental health treatment access. Even when caregiving demands necessitate reduced hours or modified roles, maintaining some degree of employment is associated with lower financial strain than complete labor force exit (Brown & Clark, 2017; Stewart et al., 2022a). National data indicate that parents providing exceptional care who remain employed experience greater economic stability and reduced vulnerability to income shocks than those who disengage entirely (Stewart et al., 2018).

Psychological Well-being, Identity, and Sense of Normalcy

Paid work can also support caregivers' psychological well-being by preserving a sense of identity beyond caregiving. Seminal qualitative studies by Rosenzweig and colleagues documented that parents of children with mental health disabilities experienced work as a domain of competence, predictability, and adult identity, particularly in contrast to the emotional intensity and uncertainty of caregiving (Rosenzweig & Huffstutter, 2004; Rosenzweig et al., 2002). Subsequent research confirms that employment can provide continuity, meaning, and a sense of normalcy amid chronic caregiving demands, particularly when work environments are stable and supportive (Sellmaier, 2019; Sellmaier & Buckingham, 2022; Stewart, 2013).

Social Connection and Reduced Isolation

Workplaces may also offer opportunities for social connection unrelated to caregiving. Parents of children with mental health conditions frequently report isolation driven by stigma and the invisibility of their child's needs (Rosenzweig et al., 2011; Sellmaier & Buckingham, 2022). In supportive organizational cultures, interactions with colleagues can provide informal emotional support and a sense of belonging that counteracts caregiving-related isolation. However, these benefits are highly contingent on workplace norms. When flexibility use is stigmatized or interpreted as diminished commitment, work-based interactions can intensify marginalization rather than alleviate it (Kossek et al., 2021).

Structure, Predictability, and Respite from Caregiving Intensity

Predictable work routines can provide temporal structure and cognitive respite in caregiving contexts marked by volatility and crisis. Parents often describe employment as a regulating force when family life is shaped by episodic mental health emergencies and uncertainty (Stewart et al., 2018). When job expectations are clear and schedules are controllable, work can reduce cognitive overload and offer relief from continuous caregiving vigilance. In contrast, unpredictable or employer-controlled schedules undermine this stabilizing function, limiting the extent to which work can serve as a source of respite (Schneider & Harknett, 2021).

Conditionality and Positive Spillover

Crucially, the positive effects of work depend on whether flexibility and support are safe to use. Early qualitative work showed that parents actively sought to remain employed because of work's protective psychological and functional role, but only when workplace conditions acknowledged caregiving realities and minimized stigma (Rosenzweig et al., 2002). Later research confirms that positive spillover from work to family life is most likely when flexibility is formalized, equitably available, and accompanied by family-supportive supervision (Hammer et al., 2011; Stewart et al., 2018). When workplaces are inflexible, stigmatizing, or organized around ideal-worker norms, employment can exacerbate strain and accelerate economic and emotional exhaustion. Under these conditions, work becomes another site of risk rather than a source of stability.

Hence, the literature reframes paid work as a potential adaptive resource rather than an inherent liability for parents raising children with mental health disabilities. When employment is secure, predictable, and supported by inclusive workplace practices, it can buffer financial risk, sustain caregiver identity, reduce isolation, and stabilize family life across cycles of crisis and reorganization. When these conditions are absent, the protective potential of work erodes, reinforcing the central argument of this chapter: work–family outcomes for parents providing exceptional care are shaped less by individual coping or commitment than by structural alignment between caregiving demands and employment contexts.

Part 7: Implications for Social Work Practice

For social workers working with parents of children with mental health disabilities employment and financial contexts are not peripheral concerns but central determinants of family stability, service access, and well-being. Parents' caregiving strategies, treatment decisions, and engagement with systems are shaped by the need to maintain income, health insurance, and job security in the face of unpredictable and intensive care demands.

First, social workers must recognize that financial strain and work disruption are structurally produced, not indicators of family dysfunction. Employment instability, reduced work hours, and income loss often reflect inflexible labor markets and fragmented service systems rather than lack of parental commitment. Practice approaches that fail to account for these constraints risk misattributing systemic barriers to individual or family-level deficits.

Second, social workers play a critical role in supporting parents' employment-related decision-making, including decisions about workplace disclosure, flexibility requests, and job changes. Parents' use of concealment or partial disclosure should be understood as risk management strategies designed to protect family income and caregiving capacity. Practice grounded in self-determination requires supporting parents to assess risks and options rather than pressuring disclosure or accommodation requests that may jeopardize economic stability.

Third, integrating employment and financial assessment into routine practice strengthens intervention planning. Understanding parents' job characteristics, access to flexibility, and exposure to financial risk allows social workers to anticipate barriers to treatment adherence, align service plans with realistic time and income constraints, advocate for accommodations within schools, healthcare systems, and workplaces, and connect families to financial, legal, and employment-related resources. Finally, this perspective reinforces social workers' advocacy role. The cumulative financial penalties experienced by families raising children with mental health disabilities reflect broader policy and labor market failures. Social workers are well positioned to translate family experiences into organizational change, policy reform, and systems-level advocacy aimed at reducing income insecurity and supporting sustainable caregiving.

Part 8: Summary and Key Points

This chapter advanced the book's central argument that parenting a child with a mental health disability is a long-term, structurally produced work–life dilemma rather than a time-limited family challenge. By conceptualizing exceptional caregiving as a chronic social condition, the chapter situated parents' experiences within the intersecting systems of work, health, and social policy that shape caregiving capacity over time.

Drawing on longitudinal, population-based, and qualitative research from the United States, the chapter demonstrated that the effects of parenting a child with mental health needs accumulate across the life course, influencing caregivers' employment trajectories, economic security, and physical and psychological health. Evidence from Seltzer and colleagues' work with aging parents of adults with serious mental illness illustrated how decades of caregiving can shape stress physiology and health into later life, while population-level studies by Witt and others showed that parents of children with activity-limiting mental health conditions experience poorer health and greater work disruption than parents of typically developing children. Together, these findings underscore that exceptional caregiving produces enduring consequences that extend well beyond childhood.

Also emphasized is the conditional role of employment. While work can exacerbate strain under inflexible or stigmatizing conditions, it can function as a protective resource when jobs are stable, predictable, and supported by family-responsive workplace practices. Under aligned conditions, employment can buffer financial risk, sustain caregiver identity, reduce isolation, and provide structure and respite amid chronic uncertainty. These outcomes, however, are shaped less by individual choice than by structural fit between caregiving demands and labor market conditions.

From a social work practice perspective, this framing underscores the need to move beyond crisis-oriented or child- or parent-only interventions. Social workers encounter parents of children with mental health disabilities across clinical, educational, and community settings, and are uniquely positioned to assess how employment conditions, economic precarity, and policy gaps intensify family stress. At micro and mezzo levels, practice can integrate work-related considerations into service planning and support families navigating disclosure and accommodation decisions. At the macro level, the chapter reinforces social work's role in advocating for policies and organizational practices that recognize exceptional caregiving as a long-term social condition.

Part 9: Application for Social Work Education

The following exercises are designed for use in undergraduate and graduate social work courses, professional training, and applied learning settings. They emphasize critical thinking, ethical reasoning, and application across micro, mezzo, and macro levels of practice.

EXERCISE 1: MAPPING WORK–CARE PRECARITY (MICRO-LEVEL PRACTICE) MAPPING WORK–CARE PRECARITY (MICRO-LEVEL PRACTICE)

Competency 7: Assess Individuals, Families, Groups, Organizations, and Communities

Competency 8: Intervene with Individuals, Families, Groups, Organizations, and Communities

Purpose

To help students recognize how employment strain emerges from structural misfit rather than individual failure.

Instructions

Ask students to select a case example from the chapter (or a composite client scenario). Have them map the client's caregiving demands against workplace expectations, identifying points of misalignment. Students should then identify how stigma, flexibility use, and financial considerations shape the client's choices.

Learning outcomes

- Apply person-in-environment analysis to employment decisions
- Distinguish coping challenges from structural constraints

EXERCISE 2: DISCLOSURE DECISION SIMULATION (ETHICS AND CLINICAL JUDGMENT) DISCLOSURE DECISION SIMULATION (ETHICS AND CLINICAL JUDGMENT)

Competency 2: Advance Human Rights and Social, Racial, Economic, and Environmental Justice

Competency 6: Engage with Individuals, Families, Groups, Organizations, and Communities

Competency 7: Assess Individuals, Families, Groups, Organizations, and Communities
Competency 8: Intervene with Individuals, Families, Groups, Organizations, and Communities

Purpose

To develop skills in supporting risk-informed decision-making without defaulting to disclosure as best practice.

Instructions

Present students with a scenario in which a parent must decide whether and how to disclose caregiving needs to an employer. Students work in small groups to identify potential risks and benefits, including short- and long-term consequences. Groups then discuss how a social worker might support the client without imposing a preferred outcome.

Learning outcomes

- Practice ethical reasoning under conditions of uncertainty
- Understand disclosure as a structurally constrained decision

EXERCISE 3: MAKING INVISIBLE LABOR VISIBLE (MEZZO-LEVEL PRACTICE) MAKING INVISIBLE LABOR VISIBLE (MEZZO-LEVEL PRACTICE)

Competency 2: Advance Human Rights and Social, Racial, Economic, and Environmental Justice
Competency 3: Engage Anti-Racism, Diversity, Equity, and Inclusion (ADEI) in Practice

Purpose

To build skills in translating caregiving labor into institutionally legible forms.

Instructions

Students identify examples of invisible caregiving labor from the chapter (anticipatory vigilance, crisis response, systems navigation). They then practice reframing these demands into functional impacts that could be communicated to schools, healthcare providers, or employers without violating privacy.

Learning outcomes

- Recognize and articulate invisible caregiving labor
- Develop advocacy-oriented communication strategies

EXERCISE 4: FINANCIAL STRAIN ACROSS THE LIFE COURSE (MACRO-LEVEL ANALYSIS) FINANCIAL STRAIN ACROSS THE LIFE COURSE (MACRO-LEVEL ANALYSIS)

Competency 5: Engage in Policy Practice

Purpose

To examine cumulative disadvantage resulting from caregiving-related employment disruption.

Instructions

Students trace how a single caregiving crisis might lead to reduced hours, benefit loss, or stalled advancement over time. They then identify policy gaps and propose interventions at organizational or legislative levels that could mitigate long-term financial risk.

Learning Outcomes

- Understand cumulative disadvantage
- Connect individual experiences to policy and labor market structures

EXERCISE 5: PRACTICE INTEGRATION REFLECTION PRACTICE INTEGRATION REFLECTION

Competency 1: Demonstrate Ethical and Professional Behavior
Competency 2: Advance Human Rights and Social, Racial, Economic, and Environmental Justice
Competency 3: Engage Anti-Racism, Diversity, Equity, and Inclusion (ADEI) in Practice

Purpose

To help students integrate learning across levels of practice.

Instructions

Ask students to reflect on how social workers can simultaneously support individual families, engage institutions, and advocate for systemic change. Students should identify one concrete action they could take at each level of practice based on the chapter's findings.

Learning Outcomes

- Integrate micro, mezzo, and macro perspectives

Resource List

Foundational Readings on Work–Care Precarity, Time, and Careers

These works provide the conceptual grounding for understanding why caregiving-related employment strain is structurally produced, rather than the result of individual choice or poor planning. Together, they illuminate how time norms, career expectations, and organizational practices shape inequality for caregivers.

- Blair-Loy, M. (2023). *Work without end: Scheduling flexibility and worker insecurity*. Russell Sage Foundation.
- Jacobs, J. A., & Gerson, K. (2004). *The time divide: Work, family, and gender inequality*. Harvard University Press.
- Moen, P. (2003). *It's about time: Couples and careers*. Cornell University Press.
- Moen, P., & Roehling, P. (2005). *The career mystique: Cracks in the American dream*. Rowman & Littlefield.
- Moen, P., & Kelly, E. L. (2020). *Overload: How good jobs went bad and what we can do about it*. Princeton University Press.
- Stone, P. (2007). *Opting out? Why women really quit careers and head home*. University of California Press.
- Gerson, K., & Damaske, S. (2021). *The science and art of balancing work and family*. Oxford University Press.

Work–Family Integration, Flexibility, and Organizational Contexts

These texts examine how workplace norms, flexibility regimes, and organizational cultures shape caregiving risk and opportunity. They are particularly relevant for understanding why flexibility may exacerbate precarity when it is informal or weakly protected.

- Kossek, E. E., & Thompson, R. J. (Eds.). (2016). *Work–life integration: Organizational, cultural, and individual perspectives*. Routledge.
- Williams, J. C., Blair-Loy, M., & Berdahl, J. L. (2016). *What works for women at work: Four patterns working women need to know*. NYU Press.

Mental Health Caregiving, Systems of Care, and Employment

This volume centers families caring for children with emotional and behavioral health needs and situates employment challenges within fragmented systems of care. It provides essential context for understanding courtesy stigma and crisis-driven caregiving.

- Rosenzweig, J. M., & Brennan, E. M. (Eds.). (2008). *Work, life, and the mental health system of care: A guide for professionals supporting families of children with emotional or behavioral disorders*. Paul H. Brookes Publishing Co.

Policy, Legal, and Practice-Oriented Web Resources

The following organizations provide applied tools, policy guidance, and legal frameworks relevant to social workers supporting families navigating employment, caregiving, and mental health systems.

Employment Protections and Legal Context

- U.S. Department of Labor, Wage and Hour Division (Family and Medical Leave Act): https://www.dol.gov/agencies/whd/fmla
- U.S. Equal Employment Opportunity Commission (EEOC): https://www.eeoc.gov
- Center for WorkLife Law, UC Law San Francisco: https://worklifelaw.org

Work–Family Research and Organizational Practice

- Families and Work Institute: https://familiesandwork.org

References

Brannan, A. M., Brennan, E. M., Sellmaier, C., & Rosenzweig, J. M. (2018). Employed parents of children receiving mental health services: Caregiver strain and work–life integration. *Families in Society, 99*(1), 29–44. https://doi.org/10.1177/1044389418756375

Brennan, E. M., Jivanjee, P., Rosenzweig, J. M., & Stewart, L. M. (2016). Challenges and supports for employed parents of children and youth with special needs. In T. Allen & L. Eby (Eds.), *Oxford Handbook of work and family* (pp. 165–181). Oxford University Press.

Brown, T. J., & Clark, C. (2017). Employed parents of children with disabilities and work family life balance: A literature review. *Child Youth Care Forum, 46*(6). https://doi.org/10.1007/s10566-017-9407-0

Clair, J. A., Beatty, J. E., & MacLean, T. L. (2005). Out of sight but not out of mind: Managing invisible social identities in the workplace. *Academy of Management Review, 30*, 78–95. https://doi.org/10.5465/amr.2005.15281431

Corrigan, P. W., & Miller, F. E. (2004). Shame, blame and contamination: A review of the impact of mental illness on family members. *Journal of Mental Health, 13*, 537–548. https://doi.org/10.1080/09638230400017004

DeRigne,L. (2012). The employment and financial effects on families raising children with special health care needs: An examination of the evidence. *Journal of Pediatric Health Care, 26*(4), 283–290. https://doi.org/10.1016/j.pedhc.2010.12.006

DeRigne, L. A., & Porterfield, S. L. (2017). Employment change among married parents of children with special health care needs. *Journal of Family Issues, 38*, 579–606. https://doi.org/10.1177/0192513X15572368

Galinsky, E., Sakai, K., & Wigton, T. (2011). Workplace flexibility: From research to action. In *The Future of Children, 21*(2), 141–161. https://doi.org/10.1353/foc.2011.0019

Goffman, E. (1963). *Stigma: Notes on the management of spoiled identity*. Prentice Hall.

Greenhaus, J. H., & Allen, T. D. (2011). Work–family balance: A review and extension of the literature. In J. C. Quick & L. E. Tetrick (Eds.), *Handbook of occupational health psychology* (2nd ed., pp. 165–183). American Psychological Association.

Hammer, L. B., Kossek, E. E., Anger, W. K., Bodner, T., & Zimmerman, K. L. (2011). Clarifying work–family intervention processes: The roles of work–family conflict and family-supportive supervisor behaviors. *Journal of Applied Psychology, 96*(1), 134–150. https://doi.org/10.1037/a0020927

Hochschild, A. R. (1997). When work becomes home and home becomes work. *California Management Review*, *39*(4), 79–97. https://doi.org/10.1177/000812569703900401

Kossek, E. E., Thompson, R. J., & Lautsch, B. A. (2021). Balanced workplace flexibility: Avoiding the traps. *California Management Review*, *63*(4), 5–25. https://doi.org/10.1525/cmr.2015.57.4.5

Lewis, S. (2003). The integration of paid work and the rest of life: Is post-industrial work the new leisure? *Leisure Studies*, *22*(4), 343–355. https://doi.org/10.1080/02614360310001594131

Lewis, S., Gambles, R., & Rapoport, R. (2007). The constraints of a 'work-life balance' approach: An international perspective. *The International Journal of Human Resource Management*, *18*(3), 360–373. https://doi.org/10.1080/09585190601165577

Parish, S. L., & Cloud, J. M. (2006). Financial well-being of young children with disabilities and their families. *Social Work*, *51*, 223–232. https://doi.org/10.1093/sw/51.3.223

Parish, S. L., Seltzer, M. M., Greenberg, J. S., & Floyd, F. (2004). Economic implications of caregiving at midlife: Comparing parents with and without children who have developmental disabilities. *Ment Retard*, *42*(6), 413–26. https://doi.org/10.1352/0047-6765(2004)42<413:EIOCAM>2.0.CO;2

Pleck, J. H. (1977). The work-family role system. *Social Problems*, *24*(4), 417–427. https://doi.org/10.1525/sp.1977.24.4.03a00040

Porterfield, S. L., & DeRigne, L. (2011). Medical home and out-of-pocket medical costs for children with special health care needs. *Pediatrics*, *128*(5), 892–900. https://doi.org/10.1542/peds.2010-1307

Ragins, B. R. (2008). Disclosure disconnects: Antecedents and consequences of disclosing invisible stigmas across life domains. *Academy of Management Review*, *33*(1), 194–215. https://doi.org/10.5465/amr.2008.27752724

Rosenzweig, J. M., Barnett, R. C., Huffstutter, K., & Stewart, L. M. (2008). Work-life integration: History, theory and strategy. In J. M. Rosenzweig & E. M. Brennan (Eds.), *Work, life, and the mental health system of care: A guide for professionals supporting families of children with emotional or behavioral disorders* (pp. 89–115). Paul H. Brookes.

Rosenzweig, J. M., Brennan, E. M., & Ogilvie, A. (2002). Work-family fit: Voices of parents of children with emotional and behavioral disorders. *Social Work*, *47*, 415–424. https://doi.org/10.1093/sw/47.4.415

Rosenzweig, J. M., Huffstutter, K., Malsch, A., Stewart, L. M. & Brennan, E. M. (2011). Voices at the table: Views of parents and human resource professionals on managing the work-family boundary. *Special Issue on Family Voices/Perspectives for Best Practices in Mental Health: An International Journal*, 7(1), 67–93.

Rosenzweig, J. M., & Huffstutter, K. M. (2004). Disclosure and reciprocity: On-the-job strategies for taking care of business…and family. *Focal Point: A National Bulletin on Family Support and Children's Mental Health*, 4–7.

Schneider, D., & Harknett, K. (2021). Hard times: Routine schedule unpredictability and material hardship among service sector workers. *Social Forces; A Scientific Medium of Social Study and Interpretation*, *99*(4), 1682–1709. https://doi.org/10.1093/sf/soaa079

Sellmaier, C. (2019). Work, family, and community ecologies and their influence on work–life fit for fathers of children with special health care needs. *Families in Society*, *100*(1), 68–79. https://doi.org/10.1177/1044389418811945

Sellmaier, C., & Buckingham, S. (2022). "I think sometimes that dads are kind of forgotten (…) so it's nice that we also get a voice.": Work-life experiences of employed U.S. fathers caring for a child with special health care needs. *Community, Work, & Family*, *25*(5), 661–676. https://doi.org/10.1080/13668803.2021.1911935

Sellmaier, C., Leo, M. C., Brennan, E. M. Kendall, J., & Houck, G. M. (2016). Finding fit between work and family responsibilities when caring for children with ADHD diagnoses. *Journal of Child and Family Studies*, 25. 3684–3693. https://doi.org/10.1007/s10826-016-0527-1

Sellmaier, C., Stewart, L. M., & Brennan, E. M. (2020). Workforce engagement of children and youth with mental health disabilities: The impact of community services and supports. *Community, Work and Family*, *23*(5), 534–555. https://doi.org/10.1080/13668803.2020.1820954

Stewart, L. M. (2009). *Dependent care and work-life outcomes: Comparing exceptional and typical care responsibilities* [Doctoral Dissertation].

Stewart, L. M. (2013). Exploring the impact of type of family care on work-family and family-work conflict. *Journal of Family Issues*, *34*(1), 113–138. https://doi.org/10.1177/0192513X12437708.

Stewart, L. M., & Charles, A. (2021). Disclose or conceal: How employees caring for dependent older adults and those caring for children with disabilities manage the communication boundaries at work. *Journal of Family Issues*, *43(*6), 1536–1554. https://doi.org/10.1177/0192513X211026965

Stewart, L. M., Sellmaier, C., Brannan, A. M. et al. (2022a). Employed parents of children with typical and exceptional care responsibilities: Family demands and workplace supports. *Journal of Child and Family Studies*, *32*, 1048–1064. https://doi.org/10.1007/s10826-022-02363-5

Stewart, L. M., Sellmaier, C., Brannan, A. M., & Brennan, E. M. (2022b). Supporting sleep and health of employed parents with typical and exceptional care demands. *Journal of Social Service Research*, *48*(2), 259–272. https://doi.org/10.1080/01488376.2021.2024935

Stewart, L. M., Sellmaier, C., Henderson-Posther, M., Lukefahr, J., & Brennan, E. M. (2025). Navigating stigma and discrimination at work while parenting a child with a mental health disability. In P. N. Claster & S. L. Blair (Eds.), *Disability and the family: Challenges, resources, and resilience* (Vol. 27, p. 0). Emerald Publishing Limited. https://doi.org/10.1108/S1530-353520250000027005

Stewart, L. M., Stutz, H., & Lile, W. (2018). Dependent care: A theoretical explanation of correlates and health consequences. *Special Issue Community, Work and Family*, *21(*5). https://doi.org/10.1080/13668803.2018.1530637

Voydanoff, P. (2007). *Work, family, and community: Exploring interconnections*. Lawrence Erlbaum Associates.

Warfield, M. E. (2005). Family and work predictors of parenting role stress among two-earner families of children with disabilities. *Infant Child Development*, *14*, 155–176. https://doi.org/10.1002/icd.386

Williams, J. C. (2000). *Unbending gender: Why family and work conflict and what to do about it*. Oxford University Press.

6

SOCIAL SUPPORT AND COMMUNITY RESOURCES

This chapter will take a closer look at the role of social support and community resources for parents trying to manage work and family responsibilities. The previous chapters discussed the challenges and opportunities related to employment and how families are impacted by exceptional care demands. In the early stages of work–family research, these were usually the only two systems included in the discussion, but over the years the field expanded to also include the broader community and its influence on the work-life continuum. In this chapter, we will examine the role of day cares and schools, medical and therapeutic services, respite care, and peer support. All families interact with day cares and schools, utilize medical services at times, and connect with other parents. Families with exceptional care responsibilities face unique challenges when interacting with these systems, which has been mentioned when discussing caregiver strain and stress in Chapter 4. Social work can play an integral role in making community resources more accessible, so that they can support families to meet work and care demands instead of increasing stress and strain on the family system. Social work's person-in-environment approach lends itself to understanding that families are involved in myriad systems, which impact their personal and family functioning and well-being.

Part 1: Research about Child Care and Schools

> So we've specifically moved close to that school, we are like 2.5 miles away so that they could go there. At first it was fairly expensive, I can't remember exactly what it was but now "name state" has passed a law the special needs scholarship where my sons go to the school now basically tuition free.
>
> There is multiple time I mean he there was for the first couple of years we were in school 2 or 3 times a week. Yep, yep, there was either behavioral issue or some

DOI: 10.4324/9781003532668-6

> other issue that was going on that we had to go to school. So that means you're not at work for that time, you know you're getting phone calls, and the schools are asking questions.
>
> I can also you know flex my schedule. So, when M. lost the daycare all of a sudden, I had no one to watch him you know certain days a week, so I just had to leave work but then I am able to come in on Saturdays.

Historic Background

Day care and schools have the responsibility to educate children, and they are also critical for families trying to raise children and maintain employment. From the beginning, early social workers were involved in issues of child welfare, which included concerns about care of children whose mothers went to work all day. In the late 1800s and early 1900s when poor women increasingly turned to factory work in urban areas, there were no established day care facilities who would care for the children during the parent's workday. Maybe there was a neighbor who was able to look after the children, or children were left at home or in the neighborhood without supervision. Early social work recognized this situation as unsustainable for child and family well-being. For example, Hull House settlement included child care provisions, but during the progressive era, the focus of social work advocacy was on implementing a financial benefit that would support widowed mothers so that they could stay at home and take care of their children. Child well-being was therefore closely linked to mothers as full-time care providers instead of arguing for better child care so that mothers could both work and care for their children. In this vein, early social work argued for prevention to reduce or eliminate the risk of losing a wage-earning husband, making the widows' pensions long-term irrelevant (Breckinridge, 1927). The first major federal legislation to publicly fund child care came with the Defense Housing and Community Facilities and Services Act or the Lanham Act of 1940. To support the war effort and defense industry, women including mothers were needed to fill those jobs with men fighting in World War II. The Lanham Act of 1940 provided funding to offer child care to all families who needed it. The services were subsidized and therefore affordable, especially since the subsidies were not means-tested or tied to a family's income. Unfortunately, these efforts were dismantled once World War II ended, arguing that mothers' contributions in the workplace were not needed anymore and that mothers were better suited to care for their children than child care centers, citing concerns about the negative effects of child care centers on children's development. Child care policies in the United States since then focused primarily on providing child care tax credits. In general, one can observe a tension between child care as primarily educational or as primarily custodial (Palley & Shdaimah, 2014). Framing child care as educational does not center the need for families to secure child care to maintain employment, and educational programming might not meet the needs of families related to work. As noted in the below quote by Cahan (1989), there also seems to be a tension between framing child care as driven by the welfare system or by the federal government.

> The administration of child care programs created in response to maternal employment patterns has fallen either to the welfare system or to the federal government. When considered a function of social welfare, child care was stigmatized by the stamp of poverty. When supported by the federal government, the provision of child care was deemed a temporary emergency measure in response to national labor crises. When the crises ended, so did public support for child care.

With the changes to Aid to Dependent Children over the years and especially with the latest iteration of changes manifesting in the Temporary Assistance to Needy Families, maternal employment for poor families is constructed as morally virtuous and beneficial for children's well-being, and child care is provided through the welfare system.

BOX 6.1 CHANGES TO WORK REQUIREMENTS

Aid to Families with Dependent Children was established in 1935 as part of the Social Security Act. This cash benefit was available to children whose parents were not able to provide for them because of disability, unemployment or death. With the passing of the 1988 Family Support Act, cash benefits were tied to mandatory work and training requirements, finalizing a shift that started already in the 1960s with first mandating treatment and case management services for recipients. Temporary Aid for Needy Families (TANF) which was established in the Personal Responsibility and Work Opportunity Reconciliation Act of 1996 ending the entitlement to welfare by establishing time limits on welfare receipt to reduce welfare dependency and move recipients into employment.

Child Care Costs

Federal and state child care subsidy schemes are also means-tested and although the income levels vary across states, on average the threshold is set at 61% of state median income (Chien, 2024) and based on federal eligibility 69% of 3-year old children below 100% of the poverty threshold received subsidies compared to 5% of 3-year old children at 200% and over of the federal poverty threshold. These benefits are also tied to parents either being employed or seeking employment (Chien, 2024). As mentioned above, otherwise families might be eligible for the Child and Dependent Care tax credit, if they work and have taxable income to claim. According to a report from Boyle et al. (2021), the average tax credit in

2018 was $586. The tax credit was temporarily increased during the COVID-19 pandemic, but since then has returned to the levels set in 2001. Since this is a credit on the amount of federal taxes owed by the family, low-income families with little federal tax liability might not receive any or very little Child and Dependent Care tax credits. According to the report, households with incomes up to $12,000 received on average $124 in tax credits, compared to households with incomes over $500,000 who received on average $611. Unfortunately, the average cost of child care in the United States greatly exceeds these average tax credits, with average annual cost being estimated at $13,128 in 2024 (Child Care Aware, 2023).

BOX 6.2 U.S. CHILD CARE COSTS

The U.S. Department of Labor's Women's Bureau has a National Database on Childcare Prices, which allows the user to examine childcare prices on the county level from 2008 to 2022. It also includes information about childcare costs as a share of the median family income in the county and other economic and demographic information. Explore this information for your county. https://www.dol.gov/agencies/wb/topics/featured-childcare

In addition to affordability, families also face barriers related to the availability and quality of child care. The issues discussed in this section are not unique to families caring for a child with a mental health disability, but they are important context to keep in mind as we discuss the more unique issues. The specific concerns play out in front of this background of a generally limited governmental response to ensuring affordable quality child care for all families.

Child Care and Disability

When looking at child care and early childhood education specifically as it relates to children with disabilities, we have to examine Head Start and Early Head Start programs. Early Head Start is geared toward families with children from birth to three years of age, and Head Start covers the preschool years from age three to five. The goal of this programming is to provide the education to prepare children for success in school and life beyond school. Head Start programs also support families through parenting support or connecting them with community resources. The focus of this federal program is on supporting low-income families, but all programs are also required to offer 10% of its enrollment to children with disabilities independent of family income. Head start programs can also play an important role in identifying disabilities or behavioral concerns and provide early intervention services directly or connect families with community-based services. Unfortunately, not all eligible families are able to secure a spot in a Head Start program, leaving many families to turn to child care services with providers who are not specifically trained to meet their children's needs. In general, parents often report concerns about the quality of care and a lack of specific knowledge or training of providers to adequately work with their child (Ceglowski et al., 2009; Mereoiu et al., 2015; Rosenzweig et al., 2008). This lack of training and knowledge can leave providers overwhelmed and increase the risk for children to be expelled from child care programs. In one qualitative study, child care providers reported receiving little training to deal proactively with difficult behaviors, to implement environmental changes to support positive behaviors, or to teach social-emotional skills (Quesenberry et al., 2014). Some also received little support from administrators. According to the Administration for Children and Families, preschool children are three times more likely to be expelled than school-aged children in grades K-12, and disability is one factor that can increase the risk for expulsions (Administration for Children & Families, 2025). They also state that behavioral concerns are the most likely cause for a child's expulsion from day care. Losing child care leaves the child without the beneficial educational experiences and without opportunities to socialize and develop peer relationships. Expulsions in early childhood might also affect the schooling experience later in the child's life (Blacher & Eisenhower, 2023). In addition, unstable child care situations leave parents without the care needed to maintain employment and consequently a lack of stable child care has been identified as one factor for reductions or disruptions of employment especially for mothers (Montes & Halterman, 2008; Sellmaier et al., 2020) and an increased level of caregiver strain due to missing out on work responsibilities (Brennan & Brannan, 2005). Parents of children with mental health disabilities might also be less likely to depend on extended family members to help with child care, since they also might feel not well-equipped to meet the requirements for providing adequate care, adding to the risk associated with losing stable child care. It is important to mention here that child care providers are required to provide reasonable accommodations for successful inclusion of children with disabilities as stipulated by the Americans with Disabilities Act (U.S. Department of Justice Civil Rights Division, n.d.). For example, staff should receive appropriate training to effectively deal with externalizing behaviors. Providers can exclude a child if the accommodations would fundamentally change the program or if the child poses a direct threat to others in the program. Decisions have to be made for each child individually, and behavior supports have to be used first before expelling a child from care. Despite these provisions, expulsions remain a concern, especially for children with behavioral issues, and parents would have to pursue legal remedies after an expulsion, which can be costly and time consuming. Specific training for providers, lower teacher-to-student ratios, overall improved work conditions, and mental health consultations are needed to make sure that child care providers can adequately accommodate children with disabilities, and children can receive stable and high-quality care (Administration for Children & Families, 2025; Brennan et al., 2002).

School and Disability

Once children grow older, they enter Kindergarten usually at age five in the United States. Section 504 of the Rehabilitation Act of 1973 provides protections against discrimination for students with disabilities in schools receiving federal funding (U.S. Department of Education, 2025). This law requires schools to provide accommodations to disabled students so that they can successfully participate in the general curriculum. The Individuals with Disabilities Education Act (IDEA) of 1975 guarantees free public education in the least restricted environment for disabled students (U.S. Department of Education, n.d.). Schools are required to develop an individualized education program (IEP) to provide individual support to students with disabilities. All students should spend as much time as possible in the general education classroom and receive inclusive education. Section 504 uses a broader definition of disability and can cover a wider range of disabilities. The IDEA requires that students fall within 13 defined diagnostic categories such as autism, emotional disturbance, or traumatic brain injury. Despite these legal provisions not all students who would qualify receive the required accommodations (DuPaul et al., 2019).

Unfortunately, students with disabilities still have lower high school graduation rates and higher rates of school discipline and expulsions despite these legal protections. According to the National Center for Education Statistics (2024), in 2022/23 74% of students covered by the IDEA graduated from high school with a regular diploma and 10% received an alternative diploma, compared to a high school graduation rates for all students at 87% in 2021/2022. Disabled students are also overrepresented in the area of discipline, since they make up 25% of out-of-school suspensions and 23% of expulsions but they only make up 13% of the whole student population in the United States (Institute of Education Sciences, 2023). Students experiencing multiple marginalization related to race or income might have even worse outcomes (Cannon et al., 2013).

In addition to ongoing concerns about the quality of education, parents also report difficulties at the intersection of school and work. For example, schools would often call parents to pick up their child at short notice due to behavioral concerns, making it difficult for parents to maintain regular full-time work schedules (Rosenzweig et al., 2002). Teachers also agreed that they needed more training to deal with externalizing behaviors and more knowledge about mental health issues (Reinke et al., 2011). Students might also miss more days of school due to their mental health needs (Brennan & Brannan, 2005), which can affect the child's overall educational trajectory as well. Another area of struggle was transportation, since children often were excluded from school buses due to behavior concerns, leaving parents as the sole means of transportation (Rosenzweig et al., 2002). After-school and summer care can be especially challenging for parents of children with mental health disabilities. They might rely on older siblings or in-home care providers to fill some of the gaps (Rosenzweig et al., 2002). Another barrier can be age restrictions with many programs not available for older children, but children with mental health

TABLE 6.1 School and Child Care Related Legislation and Federal Programs

Individuals with Disabilities Education Act (IDEA) of 1975	Federal legislation that requires early intervention and special education to children with disabilities. All children have to receive a free and appropriate public education in the least restrictive environment.
Section 504 of the Rehabilitation Act of 1973	Federal legislation that requires the provision of accommodations to provide free and appropriate education in the least restrictive environment. Broader definition of disability than the IDEA and focused on accommodation not special education.
Individualized Education Programme (IEP) or Individualized Family Service Plan (IFSP)	IEP and IFSP are written plans that document how providers will support families and children with disabilities. IFSP is developed for children ages 0–3, and IEP is for children older than 3.
Early Head Start	Early Head Start provides family and child support services for eligible pregnant women and eligible children 0–3 years of age. This program is specifically for low-income families, but children with disabilities above the income threshold can be enrolled in this program. At least 10% of available spots have to be provided to children with disabilities.
Head Start	Head Start is a preschool program available to eligible children (low-income, or homeless, or in foster care) at 3-years of age. Children with disabilities can be included even if they do not meet the income requirements. Similar to Early Head Start, 10% of spaces have to be offered to children with disabilities.

disabilities might need supervision beyond elementary or early middle-school years (Jinnah & Stoneman, 2007). Similar to the challenges related to child care for younger children, parents also shared that they worked fewer hours due to the struggles securing adequate care for school-aged children (Rosenzweig et al., 2008), and a greater number of school absences was also related to more caregiver strain due to missing work (Brennan & Brannan, 2005). Since parents have to meet employment requirements, they might also struggle to attend IEP meetings or other educational events. These difficulties might be interpreted by school personnel as a lack of care or interest in the child's education. Unfortunately, this ignores the fact that parents have multiple obligations that they try to manage and frequent calls from schools or frequent meetings to discuss school-related problems can be a substantial strain even if parents have flexible work schedules and ample sick leave.

Transition Years

In the context of education, we also want to mention the transition in young adulthood from K-12 education to post-secondary education or employment.

Schools are required to provide transition planning as part of an Individualized Education Program (IEP). This should include a transition assessment identifying a student's strengths, interests, and needs, setting measurable goals, and identification of appropriate transition services. Schools should include transition planning during IEP meetings once a student turns 16. The transition plan should identify classes that would support the student's transition including course work related to independent living skills, and coordinate connections with the adult-serving system to provide a smoother transition. All students with an IEP are eligible for pre-employment services offered by the Department of Vocational Rehabilitation. This can include job exploration, skills development related to interviewing or resume writing, and job skills training through employment in the community. Students who don't graduate with a high school diploma can receive special education services until age 21. One longitudinal study examining the National Longitudinal Transition Study data from 2003 to 2012 found that fewer parents and young adults reported in 2012 to have had conversations about their plans after high school, despite having regular IEP meetings (Liu et al., 2018). For the group of students with the designation "emotional disturbance" specifically, young adults were slightly more likely to report having developed a transition plan changing from 69 to 71%, but only 66% of parents reported having had conversations with school staff about a transition plan, which is significantly lower than the 79% in 2003 (Liu et al., 2018). Even if the number might have slightly increased for young adults with the designation of "emotional disturbance," this would still leave 29% of students without a transition plan. This might also explain why there is still a persistent gap when considering the long-term outcomes of enrollment in post-secondary education and employment. Only 34.7% of young adults with "emotional disturbances" were enrolled in post-secondary education compared to 62.6% of the general young adult population despite similar high school graduation rates (Brennan et al., 2016). When looking at types of colleges, 20.6% enrolled in a 2-year college, 23.2% in a vocational, business or technical school, and only 5.5% in a 4-year college (Newman et al., 2009). The picture is slightly better for employment outcomes. Overall, 56.8% of young people with disabilities reported being employed during the survey window compared to 66.4% of young people without a disability. When looking at the designation "emotional disturbance" specifically, the outcomes appear to be worse, with only 42.3% being employed at time of the interview and 63.4% ever since leaving high school (Newman et al., 2009). The average duration in a job for this group of young people was 7.6 months compared to 10 months for youth with any disability or 14.7 months for young people in the general population (Newman et al., 2009).

This section explored the larger historical background shaping access to child care in the U.S., showing the overall fragmented landscape of child care provisions and supports with very high cost of child care to families and limited governmental support. Despite legal restrictions of discrimination based on disability in public child care and school systems, challenges remain. Parents report difficulties finding adequate and affordable child care that can meet their child's support needs. Despite special education provisions, high school graduation rates seem to lag, and disciplinary measures are taken more frequently. Calls from schools because they are not equipped to manage a child's behavior can also disrupt parents' work schedules. After-school care or summer programs might not be available for older children, who might benefit from additional supervised activities, leaving parents with holes in care to manage themselves. Transition to adulthood can also bring unique support needs for young adults with mental health disabilities, which are not always met leading to worse outcomes related to employment and post-secondary education.

Part 2: Research about Medical and Therapeutic Services

> There are certain things that people on government benefits get like wraparound care, in-home therapies, stuff that we can't get from our private insurance, but we make too much money to be on a government plan which is kind of is unfortunate.
>
> The paperwork is too complicated, the appointments are at inconvenient times, they are too far away, yeah it's a rough path. (…) When there is a crisis her needs come up really fast, the mental health system requires prior authorization long wait times for appointments access is really hampered there is really nobody who can do any kind of in-home support so it requires taking her somewhere.
>
> Our credibility as parents (…) we are always being questioned. It's like living in a fish bowl and people ask us the same questions and it sounds like they are looking for an opportunity to say this is got to be the parents' fault. You don't get that with medical issues at least we don't get that at all but with the psyche stuff we do.

The role of medical and therapeutic care has already been mentioned in the previous chapter on the family as a system. This section will take a deeper dive into how medical services can reduce work–family conflict and caregiver strain and what obstacles remain for families interacting with the medical system.

Recent research found that across all states in the United States. 21% of parents of children with mental health concerns reported an unmet mental health need and 46% indicated difficulties in accessing mental health care (Graaf et al., 2025). There is great variability on both of those indicators across the different U.S. states. For example, 7% of parents in Montana reported unmet mental health needs compared to 32% in Utah and about 30% of parents reported difficulty accessing care in Hawaii compared to 58% in Texas. The study also confirmed discrepancies in access to care based on race, family income, and insurance status. Children identified as Black and families with lower incomes and no insurance were most likely to report unmet mental health needs (Interdepartmental Serious

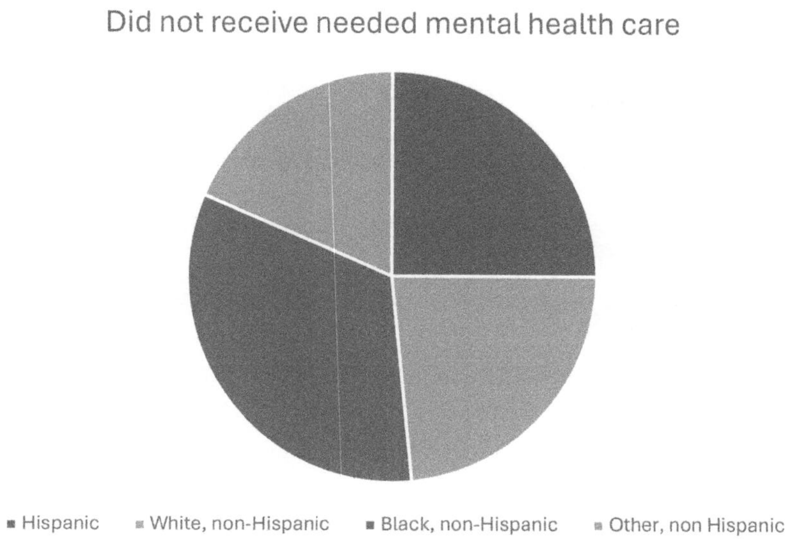

FIGURE 6.1 Unmet Mental Health Care for Different Racial Groups Based on 2023/24 National Survey of Children's Health

Mental Illness Coordinating Committee, 2022). Families without insurance were also most likely to indicate difficulties accessing care as well as children identified as Hispanic, and families with lower incomes. The authors also argue that despite changes to federal and state policies and despite investments into community mental health care, states such as Texas and California who were found

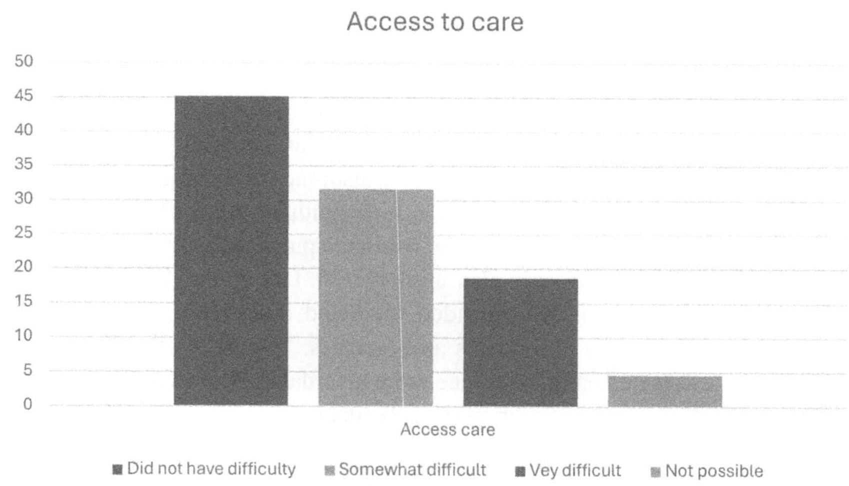

FIGURE 6.2 Difficulty Receiving Mental Health Care Based on 2023/24 National Survey of Children's Health

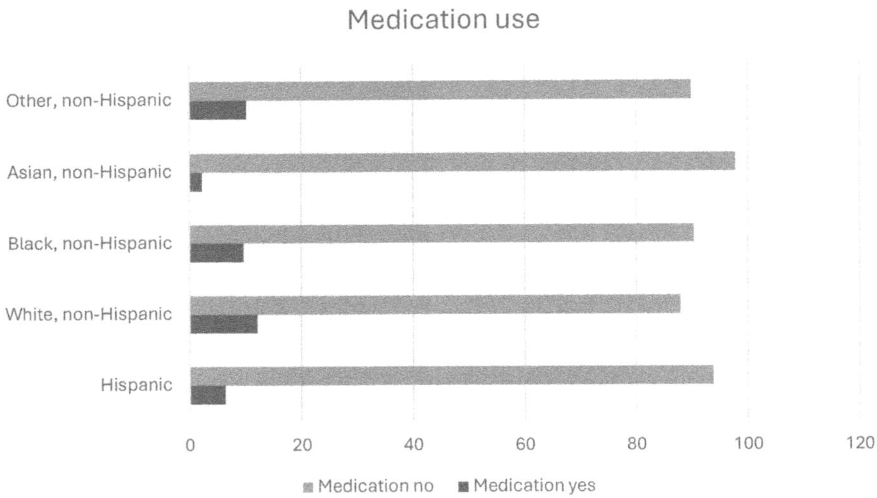

FIGURE 6.3 Medication for ADHD/ADD, ASD, or Difficulties with Emotions, Concentration, or Behavior by Race Based on 2023/24 National Survey of Children's Health

to have high unmet mental health needs in 2007, appeared to have similar difficulties in accessing health care needs in this more recent study evaluating the 2016–2019 waves of the National Survey of Children's Health. Another study analyzing 2022 data of the National Survey of Children's Health also found similar levels of unmet mental health needs (15.1%) and difficulty accessing care (59.2%; Bui et al., 2025).

Insurance

This section cannot provide a detailed analysis of the Affordable Care Act (ACA) and how it affected access to mental health care, but we would like to mention that in general with the passing of the ACA, insurance companies could not use pre-existing conditions anymore to exclude individuals from coverage, mental health care had to be covered by private insurance plans, and young adults could stay on their parents' health care plan until age 26. Due to the ACA, as of 2025 40 states and Washington DC expanded Medicaid increasing access to health insurance for low-income individuals and families. The ACA also includes tax credits to make private health insurance more affordable. The introduction of the Children's Health Insurance Program (CHIP) enacted in 1997 provided health insurance coverage to children in low-income families who did not qualify for Medicaid. Since these policy changes were enacted a drop in the child uninsured rate was found with the lowest uninsured rate of 3.9% in 2023 (Cohen et al., 2025).

Unfortunately, there has been a slight uptick again with 5.1% of U.S. children uninsured in 2024 (Cohen et al., 2025). Independent of insurance status, many mental health care providers do not accept health insurance. For example, in 2017 only 46% of psychiatrists accepted Medicaid and in 2016 only 43% accepted private health insurance plans.

Access to Medical Care

In addition to access to health insurance and the type of services covered by health insurance, a shortage especially of child and adolescent-serving mental health providers creates difficulty in accessing care. Based on information of the American Academy of Child and Adolescent Psychiatry (AACAP), there are on average 15 child and adolescent psychiatrists per 100,000 children nationally, but comparing the availability across states the number can range from 5 to 56 psychiatrists per 100,000 children (Tomopoulos & Greenblatt, 2024). In 2024, one-third of the general U.S. population, not just children, lived in a so-called mental health professional shortage area (National Center for Health Workforce Analysis, 2024). Availability of mental health care in rural areas is even more limited compared to urban areas (Woolcock et al., 2025b). For example, across the United States, there were 124.3 social workers per 100,000 people in urban areas, but only 68.6 in rural areas. These rural-urban differences also vary across U.S. states, with a 90.7–50.7 social worker difference in Washington state and a 142.9 to 69.8 urban-rural social worker difference in Illinois (Woolcock et al., 2025a, b). This provider shortage affects wait times until families can access services. The average wait time for mental health care for the general population, not children specifically, was estimated to be 48 days (National Center for Health Workforce Analysis, 2024). In 2018, the AACAP estimated the average wait time for children to meet with a psychiatrist to be 7.5 weeks (AACAP, 2018). Access to care is therefore influenced by both geographic location and individual and family characteristics such as income and race.

Experience with Medical Care

These different data points align with reports of families' experience with accessing medical care (Calderon et al., 2025; Sellmaier & Buckingham, 2022). For example, in one study parents reported that needed services were not available, that they often did not know what services to seek and that they worried about the cost of care (Hansen et al., 2021). Parents also indicated that they felt that service providers did not listen to them and did not take them seriously, at times they even felt blamed for the child's mental health disability. Children with a mental health diagnosis reported similar experiences, feeling small when working with providers and fearing stigmatization, which made them reluctant to seek care (Gotting et al., 2025). Stigmatization not just by providers but the fear of being stigmatized by others or the child experiencing negative repercussions for having a record of a mental health concern also kept parents from seeking help. The attitudes of parents toward mental health care also kept children and youth from seeking care themselves (Gotting et al., 2025). A Canadian study examining the experience of immigrant parents confirmed findings of financial barriers to services, fear of stigmatization, feeling unheard, lacking information, and facing language barriers (Tulli et al., 2020). One narrative study in the UK provided insights into the interaction of parents and the healthcare system across the diagnostic course (Harden, 2005). In the early stages of evaluation to find a diagnosis, medical care played a critical role in providing the diagnosis and the explanation for a child's behaviors and changes. This was a difficult process, since at times a parent's initial concerns were dismissed as normal teenage behavior and because finding a diagnosis was often a lengthy process. Even if a diagnosis was received, the causes and the treatment often remained elusive. Not knowing what caused a condition left parents without a clear answer what to do to support their child. Parents also reported that providers might cite parenting behaviors as a reason for the child's mental health condition. Even if providers did not blame parents, parents blamed themselves for the child's condition. Parents also had to negotiate a changed landscape of care responsibilities with medical providers now providing some of the care they traditionally provided to their own child. This was especially evident if children had to be hospitalized for treatment, leaving parents feeling like they were abandoning their children and leaving them in a place that did not always look safe. If children received out-patient care, parents were also often left outside the treatment, especially if children were old enough to consent to their own care. In the U.S. laws on consent to mental health care vary by state (Sharko et al., 2022) with many states having no explicit law on age for consent, in states with explicit laws the age varied from 12 to 16 years. Some states distinguished between in-patient and out-patient care, and some had specific stipulations for medications. This legal framework at times conflicted with the parents' experience of their child needing more care than other teenagers their age especially during a time of crisis. This is not to argue that adolescents should not have privacy protections as they seek mental health care or to undermine the benefits of privacy for building a trusting relationship, but to show that this situation can leave parents in limbo negotiating their new role in providing care and the boundaries of their ability to provide the supports their child might need. Help from providers for parents to figure out their place in this constellation of therapist, child, and parent could be beneficial. Children also reported that they valued independence in their treatment planning with the support of parents and providers (Gotting et al., 2025). A study interviewing mothers of children with ASD and a mental health condition shared similar observations, stating that they blamed themselves for their child's condition and at times were also blamed by the service provider (Jackson et al., 2019). They also reported waiting for a long time to receive mental health services and current mental health service delivery models not fitting well with their child's needs as related to ASD and mental health.

In summary, access to mental health care can be difficult, and many children do not receive adequate care in a timely manner. A lack of providers, long waiting times, and the cost of care or the lack of coverage by health insurance can create instrumental barriers to care. Stigmatization of mental health needs in general and by providers specifically, in addition to feeling unheard or not taken seriously can also hamper experience with mental health care. Blaming oneself for the condition and re-negotiating one's role as parent and carer also affects the relationship with providers. These challenges seem to be experienced by parents across different demographic variables, but there might be unique factors as well. For example, language barriers or specific therapies due to comorbidities can add further to the difficulties in accessing care. Race, education, and income also shape the service experience as well as geographic location at least in the United States. Age of the child can also increase the risk for service loss. This window when young adults move from child-serving to adult-serving systems has been described as a service cliff, since young adults often do not make this transition successfully and fall out of service receipt.

Part 3: Peer Support

> My wife has taken part-time jobs in the field before she's worked for parent advocacy agencies. We both have tried to find work where we get paid to help people in situations like we're in while also learning all the ins and outs of the system that we can apply to our own family I think that (…) some of the benefits that we've gotten out of the medical field we wouldn't have known that we were eligible for if we kind of didn't fight the good fight and used the right language.

> I would end up getting you know parenting advice, suggestions you know like take a parenting class you know you're kind of a therapist why is your kid having trouble you know what's wrong with you? Over the years I've found support from agencies like NAMI, which I think are just fantastic, given me the language to use to talk to friends, family, neighbors, employers about my situation

> We just finished a parent to parent class and we developed some friendships that was real support at that time.

In this section discussing community resources, we would also like to discuss peer support. In Chapter 4, we examined how social support by friends and extended family members might be affected by exceptional care responsibilities and what role family and friends can play in supporting families. This section will look at formal and informal peer support acknowledging that there might be overlaps between individuals showing up as friends and as peers. Peer support can be conceptualized as support from individuals with lived experience in the mental health system. Peers could be utilized for children and adolescents with mental health disabilities and for families and siblings who live with someone with a mental health issue. Given the focus of the book, we will center the discussion on family and sibling support, but peer support can also be a critical tool for the child with mental health disability. Peer support has been around for a long time with peer support practices being reported in 18th-century France and the middle of the 19th century in England (Shalaby & Agyapong, 2022). Self-help groups and organizing against involuntary confinement have also been reported in Germany in the late 19th century. Consumers and survivors of the mental health system organized in the 1960s/1970s in the United States to advocate against institutionalization and to work toward community integration and community-based services. The rallying cry "Nothing about us without us" is a reflection of this central role of people with lived experience when developing policies or conceptualizing services. Peer support became a more integrated part of service delivery in the 1990s as part of the community-based service delivery model and in 2007 peer support was considered for Medicaid reimbursement (Shalaby & Agyapong, 2022) and 41 U.S. states offer Medicaid reimbursement for both mental health and substance use peer support (Policy Center for Maternal Mental Health, 2024).

Family support services or family peer support use the experience of other parents to help families navigate the mental health care system and the general care experience. As we discussed above, parents often feel overwhelmed when interacting with the medical system, trying to figure out what services to use and how to access these services. Parents with previous experience can be a helpful resource providing information, advocacy skills, and an open ear to listen to the challenges and struggles. Family peer support can be delivered in a variety of different ways ranging from ongoing in-person or virtual family support groups, or time-limited training programs focusing on different topics such as education about mental illness, parenting skills, or coping skills. Some programs might also be delivered in collaboration with a professional provider or as part of a wraparound team (Acri et al., 2017). Peer advocates who are part of the wraparound team might provide one-on-one services dependent on the individual needs of the family, such as transportation, attending meetings, preparing families for meetings, help with forms and with understanding information (Davis et al., 2010). Research about the effectiveness of peer support is mixed (Acri et al., 2017). Shilling et al. (2013) conducted a literature review and found that in qualitative studies parents reported a sense of connection and mutual support, personal growth, and an increase in knowledge. Results from quantitative studies measuring the impact on parents' psychological well-being were mixed and only one study was found that measured the impact on service use finding weak evidence for an increase of service use for parents who received peer support. Similar mixed findings were reported in a more recent literature review (Acri et al., 2017) with some studies showing an increase in knowledge about mental health, an increase in family function and parenting skills, and a reduction in parenting concerns, but no effect on parenting stress. It is also important to mention that both reviews only found a small number of evaluation studies further limiting the evidence base about what type of peer support is most effective and in what way peer support might help families. Despite these limitations, parents themselves have reported the benefit and value of connecting with other parents with similar experiences demonstrating that these formal or informal peer connections can play a vital rŏle for families. For example, one study evaluated peer group programs one for parents and one for siblings (Feriante et al., 2022). The majority of parents reported being very satisfied with the group, appreciating connecting with parents with shared experiences, and that they learned about new resources to pursue. They also indicated that they better understand the sibling's experience, and that they had some new tools to connect. The majority of siblings also thought that it was helpful to talk to other siblings with similar experience and more siblings felt positive after the group ended than before. Peer support can therefore be considered a supportive tool for parents, siblings, and the child with mental health disability. Many parents also became peer advocates themselves, finding meaning in sharing their experience and helping other families navigate the exceptional care experience. Providing peer support can therefore be another facet of the positive impact of peer support. In addition to these more formal offerings of peer support, parents have also reported finding connection with other parents with exceptional care responsibilities in their churches, schools, and daycares, and other natural networks. Online discussion groups have also been discussed as an important venue for exchanging information and feeling a sense of connection. In one study interviewing fathers, they shared that online networks were often easier to maintain when managing a busy work and family schedule (Sellmaier & Buckingham, 2022). They also shared that support groups were more heavily frequented by mothers, which at times made it harder for them to experience this sense of connection. Groups specifically geared toward fathers were helpful, but finding time was still often a barrier.

Part 4: Respite Care

> One of the services we don't get there is no paid respite, health insurance doesn't pay for that. We really couldn't find a babysitter, so it's been a real strain on our marriage. I mean financially and physically exhausted.

> Through the waiver services he qualifies for a thing called community choice options which is something the Medicaid money can go straight to the worker that I choose to hire they just have to pass a background check and have a driver's license and what not. (…) You can't go to work when you use respite. There is a rule about that and then so that's kind of like oh I can use these respite hours

> to go get drunk which I would never do but you know you could, but I can't use respite hours to be a productive citizen and go to work you know. That doesn't make sense.

Respite refers to short-term care provided at home or in the community to offer the full-time carer a break. Respite care could be used on a regular basis or in times of crisis. The goal of respite care as an opportunity for self-care and recovery is to avoid institutionalization and to stabilize both parent and child. Respite can be provided informally by a neighbor, friend, or family member or formally through respite services. Formal respite care can include payments for neighbors or friends, as well as the use of professionals. Some U.S. states also allow that the funding can be used to pay the parent directly (Agarwal, 2025). Parents also reported acquiring certificates or licensing for example as home health aides to receive payment for some of their care work. This was especially relevant if a mother decided or was forced to give up employment to meet care responsibilities. As discussed in chapter 4, family and friends might not feel comfortable to step in as care providers, or might not be available, making formal respite care an important aspect of support for families. Paying for respite care is of course one central question for families. In the United States., respite care might be funded through two main streams, one being Medicaid waiver programs and another being vouchers through the Lifespan Respite Care program. If a child needs respite care, Medicaid waivers are often available independent of the family's income, but most states have stipulations in terms of what types of disabilities are covered. Developmental and intellectual disabilities appear to be covered by most states, but not all states have explicit coverage of mental health disabilities. Some states' programs include statements that children with disabilities other than I/DD might be eligible without further defining disability. Medicaid waiver programs also include level of care criteria usually making respite care available to families whose children require the level of care provided in a psychiatric hospital or nursing facility (Institute for Families in Society, 2019). Reviewing 2019 materials, it appears that only 11 states explicitly provided respite waivers for social-emotional disabilities (Institute for Families in Society, 2019). Families who are not eligible for respite care through the Medicaid waiver program could apply for a voucher through the Lifespan Respite Care program. This program is more open and covers anyone with a special condition that requires 40 or more hours of care or supervision, who do not receive Medicaid provided respite, and who cannot afford to pay out-of-pocket. Due to funding restrictions not all families who are eligible can receive this voucher. For example, Washington state prioritizes families who have not received a voucher before (Informing Families, n.d.), resulting in a program that families cannot rely on from year to year. Funding respite, orienting oneself in a maze of different programs with differing eligibility criteria, and meeting the eligibility criteria for a program are barriers encountered by families.

BOX 6.3 CASE EXAMPLE

Fred is a single father of 10-year-old Simon who was diagnosed with Autism. Fred works as a therapist and has some flexibility at work. Simon's child care center, which he attended before and after school was recently restructured, and Simon was not eligible to attend anymore. Fred was able to move some appointments to the weekend, so he could pick up Simon directly from school. Simon also has an intellectual disability, which makes him eligible for a Medicaid waiver and a case worker. With the help of the case worker, Fred was able to find a home health aid, paid for by the Medicaid waiver, who helps care for Simon after school. Fred would not have known how to manage Simon's after-school care long-term, if he did not qualify for the waiver program, since he couldn't have adjusted his work schedule for a longer period of time and since he doesn't have family members or friends who could have picked up Simon from school.

Even if a family receives the waiver or the voucher, it can be an issue to find qualified respite workers in the first place or replacement support should a worker leave or get sick. Usually, it takes time for a trusting relationship between respite worker and child and parents to develop and frequent changes or inconsistencies can undermine this relationship. Parents have shared the difficulty to trust another person with the care of their child, which can leave them reluctant to seek respite care at all. Accordingly, 75% of families caring for a child reported unmet respite needs (Kalman Rupp et al., 2005/06). Families also report restrictions on how respite can be used. For example, one dad shared that he can use his respite to go shopping, but he cannot use it to go to work. These restrictions at times limited the usefulness of respite for individual families. Parents have also shared that respite care that is affordable, reliable, and of high quality can be that much-needed break from ongoing care responsibilities that helps them come back with renewed energy. It can be a time for parents to reconnect and especially in community settings a time for the child with a mental health disability to connect with other children, offering a break for all family members.

Part 5: Summary and Key Points

Community resources and supports play a critical role in supporting families to meet their exceptional care responsibilities, to maintain employment and to thrive (Sellmaier & Buckingham, 2022; Sellmaier, 2019, 2021). Child care can provide developmentally important care that also helps parents to sustain a job. Schools can educate children with mental health needs and can provide the care for parents to go to work. Mental health care is of course critical for the well-being of children while also reducing exceptional care demands. Respite care can step in to provide a break for parents and offer nurturing activities for kids. Community resources therefore should be included when considering how to best support families with exceptional care demands. Unfortunately, barriers to accessing these services and programs remain. For example, the cost for child care in the United States can amount to as much as paying for college. Child care providers have to offer reasonable accommodations, but behavior concerns are one of the most cited reasons for preschool children to be expelled from care with preschool children facing higher expulsion rates than children in K-12 education. Students with disabilities might also have lower high school graduation rates and face higher rates of discipline in school. Frequent calls from schools to parents can disrupt a parent's ability to maintain employment and exclusion from bus transportation can add a demand on parent's time to drive their child to and from school. Access to mental health care can also be challenging with many reporting unmet mental health needs and difficulty accessing care. Insurance barriers and a lack of qualified mental health providers especially also in rural areas are factors contributing to these difficulties. The process itself can also be challenging for parents who might blame themselves or be blamed by providers for their child's mental health disability. Changes in care responsibilities and a lack of communication with parents can make this a difficult relationship. Funding is the main barrier to respite care in addition to a lack of qualified personnel to meet the demand.

- Community services and programs are important for supporting family resilience and help parents meet exceptional care demands.
- Barriers to accessing quality child care, K-12 education, mental health care, and respite care remain, such as lack of funding or high cost of services, lack of qualified providers and trained personnel, lack of information, and stigmatization.
- Formal and informal peer support for children with mental health disabilities, parents, and siblings can offer emotional and instrumental support for all family members.

Part 6: Recommendations for Social Work Practice

Considering the importance of community supports and the barriers that still exist, social work practitioners can play a critical role at increasing access. When thinking about improving mental health care access for children, social work advocacy can support universal health insurance to ensure coverage for all individuals. Coverage for mental health care should be provided by all insurance providers and all types of insurance plans. Advocacy for loan forgiveness programs to incentivize practitioners to specialize in mental health care for children or in rural areas can be a tool to increase the pool of providers.

When providing direct services to children with mental health needs, it is critical to provide all necessary information about the diagnosis to all family members as is permissible considering age of consent and considering the impact on the therapeutic relationship. In addition, therapeutic support should be offered to parents and siblings and in alignment with a family resilience approach, families should not be assessed as dysfunctional but as capable of adaptation. Assessing family strengths including access to community services and peer/social supports would be one important building block to support families in their adaptive process. Based on this assessment, social workers can help building linkages to support networks and other community systems, including peer support. Families participating in therapy that did not focus on parenting skills alone but checked in with parents about their own health or job concerns were less likely to drop out than families in standard therapeutic approaches (Prinz & Miller, 1994). Families who dropped out of services also reported more family adversity making regular check-ins even more crucial for success. These check-ins can be readily added to therapeutic approaches improving family and child outcomes, since they increase the likelihood that children remain in therapy.

In order to increase access to mental health care, further expansion of mental health interventions in schools and child care centers is warranted. One systematic review found that targeted and selective interventions can have a large to medium effect on reducing especially externalizing problems and even universal interventions were found to have a significant albeit small effect in elementary school settings (Sanchez et al., 2018). School social workers are well equipped to provide these types of interventions. They are also especially well situated to work with the whole family, assuring that parents and siblings are also supported and connected with community resources. Wrap-around services within a system of care can be an effective tool to provide this holistic support to the entire family system and have been found to reduce mental health symptoms and improve school outcomes (National Wraparound Initiative, 2024; Olson et al., 2021), and family members also reported behavioral improvements and better school outcomes (Brennan et al., 2016).

In addition to these improvements to mental health care, social workers can also provide more services directly geared toward parents trying to integrate work and family responsibilities. For example, disclosure in the workplace might be necessary to access workplace flexibility in times of a crisis. Social workers can assist parents in assessing their workplace, family, and community resources and demands and help parents to come to a decision about the best disclosure path based on this assessment. Providing information about available family supportive policies, such as Family Medical Leave or protections against family responsibility discrimination, can be useful as well.

- Advocacy to improve mental health care and respite access and increase providers working with children and youth.
- Continued implementation of evidence-based practices such as wraparound services in systems of care or school-based mental health services.

- Working with the whole family including parents, siblings, grandparents, and other family members or friends involved with exceptional care responsibilities. Assessing family's strengths and connecting them with relevant community services including peer support.
- Specific services to help with integration of work and exceptional care responsibilities, such as workplace disclosure support.

Part 7: Application for Social Work Education

The following activities provide ideas for working with this chapter's information both on a macro and micro level in a variety of courses.

ACTIVITY 1: POLICY ACTIVITY

Competency 2: Advance Human Rights and Social, Racial, Economic, and Environmental Justice
Competency 5: Engage in Policy Practice

Students research current provisions for coverage and reimbursement rates for mental health care for families with

- Medicaid insurance
- Private insurance

Students compare coverage between private plans and Medicaid coverage and based on type of private plan (bronze, silver, gold, platinum, or Exclusive Provider Organization, Health Maintenance Organization, Point of Service, Preferred Provider Organization)

Students can present their findings, discuss the similarities and differences, and identify potential barriers for families.

Based on the collected information on health care coverage of mental health care students develop a policy proposal or legislative ask. Students organize an advocacy campaign including letters/emails to their legislators, Take-5 tables with educational materials and information on how others can get involved, or social media campaigns.

Based on the collected information about health care coverage, students conduct a policy analysis of the Medicaid program, answering the following questions:

- What benefit/service is provided by the program?
- Who is eligible for the benefit?
- How is the program financed?
- Who implements the program?

- Does it reach the intended population, especially when considering the needs of children with mental health disabilities?
- Is everyone covered adequately, especially when considering mental health needs?
- How do the costs compare to the benefits?
- Are there unintended consequences?
- Is it aligned with social justice?

Students could conduct a policy analysis of IDEA, Early Head Start, or Head Start programs or their state's provisions of respite care as alternatives to examining Medicaid. These activities might be especially suitable to graduate students.

ACTIVITY 2: EDUCATIONAL OUTCOMES

Competency 2: Advance Human Rights and Social, Racial, Economic, and Environmental Justice

Competency 3: Engage Anti-Racism, Diversity, Equity, and Inclusion (ADEI) in Practice

Students collect graduation information and rates of suspensions and expulsions for their school district or for different states and compare these outcomes across different groups of students.

- Do they find differences across school districts or states?
- Do they find differences for these outcome measures for different student groups, i.e., students with IEP, students with 504 plan, students of different racial groups, foster care students and other groups?
- Why do they think these differences exist?
- What could social work do to address these disparities?
- If you were a school social worker, how would you support children and families with mental health disabilities?

ACTIVITY 3: UNDERSTANDING RESEARCH ABOUT COMMUNITY SERVICES

Competency 4: Engage in Practice-Informed Research and Research-Informed Practice

Competency 9: Evaluate Practice with Individuals, Families, Groups, Organizations, and Communities

Share an evaluation study about the impact of peer support or the effectiveness of wraparound services, such as the family survey report provided by the National Wraparound Initiative https://nwi.pdx.edu/pdf/nwi-telehealth-survey-family-supplement.pdf. Students discuss the following questions to grow as informed consumers of research:

- What was the sampling strategy? Who was included in the sample?
- How does this sampling influence the generalizability and validity of the findings?
- What was the data collection method and analysis strategy?
- How did data collection and data analysis influence the validity, trustworthiness, and generalizability of the findings?
- Discuss how the findings can be applied to social work practice and what limitations might exist.

ACTIVITY 4: COMMUNITY ASSESSMENT

Competency 7: Assess Individuals, Families, Groups, Organizations, and Communities
Competency 8: Intervene with Individuals, Families, Groups, Organizations, and Communities

Students conduct a community assessment of their neighborhood/town/city and gather information about

- # mental health care providers working with children including their openings and the availability of insurance-covered services
- Organizations that provide respite care, # of providers and availability
- Peer support organizations or self-help groups for individual child, parents, or siblings
- Availability of leisure time activities for child with mental health disability

Comparing different neighborhoods or towns or rural and urban areas can provide additional insights into issues of equity and justice.

Students develop an intervention plan for increasing or changing services in their assessment area based on their findings.

Resource List

Family-Run Executive Director Leadership Association: https://www.fredla.org/
National Alliance on Mental Illness: https://www.nami.org/
National Alliance on Mental Illness: Family support group: https://www.nami.org/Support-Education/Support-Groups/NAMI-Family-Support-Group/
National Federation of Families: https://www.ffcmh.org/
National Federation of Families: Peer support toolkits https://www.ffcmh.org/toolkits
National Wraparound Initiative: https://nwi.pdx.edu/

References

Acri, M., Hooley, C. D., Richardson, N., & Moaba, L. B. (2017). Peer models in mental health for caregivers and families. *Community Mental Health Journal*, *53*(2), 241–249. https://doi.org/10.1007/s10597-016-0040-4

Administration for Children & Families (2025). Understanding and eliminating expulsion in early childhood programs. Retrieved from: https://headstart.gov/publication/understanding-eliminating-expulsion-early-childhood-programs

Agarwal, S. (2025). Paid parent caregiving information. *Kid's waivers*. Retrieved from: https://www.kidswaivers.org/paid-parent-caregiving/

American Academy of Child and Adolescent Psychiatry (AACAP). (2018). Addressing children's mental health workforce shortage. Retrieved from: https://www.aacap.org/app_themes/aacap/docs/advocacy/advocacy_day/workforce_2018.pdf

Blacher, J., & Eisenhower, A. (2023). Preschool and child-care expulsion: Is it elevated for autistic children? *Exceptional Children*, *89*(2), 178–196. https://doi.org/10.1177/00144029221109234

Boyle, C. F., Crandall-Hollick, M. L., & McDermott, B. (2021). Child and dependent care tax benefits: How they work and who receives them. *Budget, Public Finance & Taxation; Education; Social Welfare Report.* Retrieved from: https://www.congress.gov/crs-product/R44993

Breckinridge, S. P. (1927). Widows' and Orphans' pensions in Great Britain. *Social Services Review*, *1*(2), 249–257. https://www.jstor.org/stable/30009038

Brennan, E. M., Ama, S. M., & Gordon, L. J. (2002). Inclusion of children with emotional or behavioral challenges in child care settings: An observational study. Retrieved from: https://pathwaysrtc.pdx.edu/pdf/pbHeadStart02.pdf

Brennan, E. M., & Brannan, A. M. (2005). Participation in the paid labor force by caregivers of children with emotional and behavioral disorders. *Journal of Emotional and Behavioral Disorders*, *13*(4), 237–246. https://doi.org/10.1177/10634266050130040501

Brennan, E. M., Nygren, P., Stephens, R. L., & Croskey, A. (2016). Predicting positive education outcomes for emerging adults in mental health systems of care. *The Journal of Behavioral Health Services & Research*, *43*(4), 564–581. https://doi.org/10.1007/s11414-015-9454-y

Bui, A. L., Ball, A. M., Ko, L. K., Ng, M., Rivara, F. P., & Coker, T. R. (2025). Foregone preventive care and unmet mental healthcare needs among U.S. youth. *American Journal of Preventive Medicine*, *69*(2), 107644. https://doi.org/10.1016/j.amepre.2025.107644

Cahan, E. (1989). Past caring: A history of U.S. preschool care and education for the poor, 1820–1965. *National Center for Children in Poverty: Mailman School of Public Health Columbia University.* Retrieved from: https://researchconnections.org/sites/default/files/pdf/rc2088.pdf

Calderon, V., Gamarra, J. M., Ruiz-Yu, B., Denenny, D. M., Zinberg, J. L., Bearden, C. E., & Miklowitz, D. J. (2025). Navigating the maze: Caregiver perspectives on pathways to mental health care for U.S. youth at clinical high risk for psychosis. *Early Intervention in Psychiatry*, *19*(3). https://doi.org/10.1111/eip.70025

Cannon, Y., Gregory, M., & Waterstone, J. (2013). A solution hiding in plain sight: Special education and better outcomes for students with social, emotional, and behavioral challenges. *The Fordham Urban Law Journal*, *41*(2), 451.

Ceglowski, D. A., Logue, M. E., Ullrich, A., & Gilbert, J. (2009). Parents' perceptions of child care for children with disabilities. *Early Childhood Education Journal*, *36*, 497–504. https://doi.org/10.1007/s10643-009-0309-0

Chien, N. (2024). Estimates of child care subsidy eligibility & receipt for fiscal year 2021. *Office of Human Services Policy.* Retrieved from: https://aspe.hhs.gov/sites/default/files/documents/a91fd97aa80b53fa52a52d38cd323509/cy2021-child-care-subsidy-eligibility.pdf#:~:text=eligibility%20parameters%20to%20set%20income%20 eligibility%20thresholds%2C,three%2Dperson%20family%20across%20all%20states%20and%20D.C.

Child Care Aware of America (2024). Child care in America: 2024 price and supply. Retrieved from: https://www.childcareaware.org/price-landscape24/

Cohen, R. A., Briones, E. M., & Inderbir Sohi, I. (2025). Health insurance coverage: Early release of estimates from the National Health Interview Survey, 2024. *National Center for Health Statistics.* Retrieved from: https://www.cdc.gov/nchs/data/nhis/earlyrelease/insur202506.pdf

Davis, T. S., Scheer, S. D., Gavazzi, S. M., & Uppal, R. (2010). Parent advocates in children's mental health: Program implementation processes and considerations. *Administration and Policy in Mental Health and Mental Health Services Research, 37*(6), 468–483. https://doi.org/10.1007/s10488-010-0288-x

DuPaul, G. J., Chronis-Tuscano, A., Danielson, M. L., & Visser, S. N. (2019). Predictors of receipt of school services in a national sample of youth with ADHD. *Journal of Attention Disorders, 23*(11), 1303–1319. https://doi.org/10.1177/1087054718816169

Feriante, J., Shayani, A., Lauer, E., Pressman, A., & Rubin, E. (2022). Sibling support program: A novel peer support intervention for parents, caregivers and siblings of youth experiencing mental illness. *Healthcare, 10*, 908. https://doi.org/10.3390/healthcare10050908

Gotting, E. K., Darcy, L., Israelsson-Skogsberg, Å., Sundler, A. J., & Lalloo, E. C. (2025). Children's experiences of living with their mental ill-health - a scoping review. *International Journal of Qualitative Studies on Health and Well-Being, 20*(1). https://doi.org/10.1080/17482631.2025.2501682

Graaf, G., Hughes, P. M., Gigli, K. H., deJong, N. A., McGrath, R. E., & Thomas, K. C. (2025). State differences in children's mental health care. *Academic Pediatrics, 25*(2), 102585. https://doi.org/10.1016/j.acap.2024.09.009

Hansen, A. S., Telléus, G. K., Mohr-Jensen, C., & Lauritsen, M. B. (2021). Parent-perceived barriers to accessing services for their child's mental health problems. *Child and Adolescent Psychiatry and Mental Health, 15*(4), 1–11. https://doi.org/10.1186/s13034-021-00357-7

Harden, J. (2005). Parenting a young person with mental health problems: Temporal disruption and reconstruction. *Sociology of Health & Illness, 27*(3), 351–371. https://doi.org/10.1111/j.1467-9566.2005.00446.x

Informing Families (n.d.). Pathways to respite. Retrieved from: https://www.dshs.wa.gov/sites/default/files/ALTSA/tbi/documents/Pathways-to-Respite.pdf

Institute for Families in Society (2019). Medicaid waivers for respite support state-by-state summaries of Medicaid waiver information. Retrieved from: https://archrespite.org/wp-content/uploads/2022/04/Medicaid_Waivers_for_Respite_2019.pdf

Institute of Education Sciences (2023). Behavior and school discipline for students with disabilities. Retrieved from: https://ies.ed.gov/learn/blog/behavior-and-school-discipline-students-disabilities

Interdepartmental Serious Mental Illness Coordinating Committee (2022). Advances through collaboration: Federal action for a system that works for all people living with SMI and SED and their families and caregivers. https://www.samhsa.gov/sites/default/files/meeting/documents/ismicc-report-to-congress-04012022.pdf

Jackson, L., Keville, S., & Ludlow, A. K. (2019). Mothers' experiences of accessing mental health care for their child with an autism spectrum disorder. *Journal of Child and Family Studies, 29*, 534–545. https://doi.org/10.1007/s10826-019-01662-8

Jinnah, H. A., & Stoneman, Z. (2007). Parents' experiences in seeking child care for school age children with disabilities—Where does the system break down? *Children and Youth Services Review, 30*, 967–977. https://doi.org/10.1016/j.childyouth.2007.11.020

Kalman Rupp, P. S., Davies, C. N., Iams, H., Becker, C., Mulpuru, S., Ressler, S., Romig, K., & Miller, B. (2005/2006). A profile of children with disabilities receiving SSI: Highlights from the National Survey of SSI Children and Families. *Social Security Bulletin, 66*(2), 21–48.

Liu, A. Y., Lacoe, J., Lipscomb, S., Haimson, J., Johnson, D. R., & Thurlow, M. L. (2018). Preparing for life after high school: The characteristics and experiences of youth in special education. Findings from the National Longitudinal Transition Study 2012. Volume 3: Comparisons over time (Executive Summary) (NCEE 2018-4008). Washington, DC: U.S. Department of Education, Institute of Education Sciences, National Center for Education Evaluation and Regional Assistance. Retrieved from: https://ies.ed.gov/sites/default/files/migrated/nces_pubs/ncee/pubs/20184007/pdf/20184008.pdf

Mereoiu, M., Bland, C., Dobbins, N., & Niemeyer, J. A. (2015). Exploring perspectives on child care with families of children with autism. *Early Childhood Research & Practice*, *17*(1).

Michel, S. (2011). The history of child care in the U.S. *VCU Libraries Social Welfare History Project.* Retrieved from: https://socialwelfare.library.vcu.edu/programs/child-care-the-american-history/

Montes, G., & Halterman, J. S. (2008). Child care problems and employment among families with preschool-aged children with autism in the United States. *Pediatrics (Evanston)*, *122*(1), e202–e208. https://doi.org/10.1542/peds.2007-3037

National Center for Education Statistics. (2024). Students with disabilities. *Condition of Education.* U.S. Department of Education, Institute of Education Sciences. Retrieved from https://nces.ed.gov/programs/coe/indicator/cgg.

National Center for Health Workforce Analysis. (2024). State of the behavioral health workforce. Retrieved from: https://bhw.hrsa.gov/sites/default/files/bureau-health-workforce/state-of-the-behavioral-health-workforce-report-2024.pdf

National Wraparound Initiative (2024). Wraparound research summary. Retrieved from: https://nwi.pdx.edu/pdf/wraparound-research-summary-10-2024.pdf

Newman, L., Wagner, M., Cameto, R., & Knokey, A.-M.. (2009). The post-high school outcomes of youth with disabilities up to 4 years after high school. A report from the National Longitudinal Transition Study-2 (NLTS2). Menlo Park, CA: SRI International. Retrieved from: https://www.nlts2.org/reports/2009_04/nlts2_report_2009_04_complete.pdf

Olson, J. R., Benjamin, P. H., Azman, A. A., Kellogg, M. A., Pullmann, M. D., Suter, J. C., & Bruns, E. J. (2021). Systematic review and meta-analysis: Effectiveness of wraparound care coordination for children and adolescents. *Journal of the American Academy of Child & Adolescent Psychiatry*, *60*(11), 1353–1366. https://doi.org/10.1016/j.jaac.2021.02.022.

Palley, E., & Shdaimah, C. S. (2014). *In our hands: The struggle for U.S. Child care policy*. New York University Press.

Policy Center for Maternal Mental Health. (2024, July). Gaps in peer support reimbursement and certification in the United States [Fact Sheet]. https://doi.org/10.69764/MTOA3221

Prinz, R. J., & Miller, G. E. (1994). Family-based treatment for childhood antisocial behavior: Experimental influences on dropout and engagement. *Journal of Consulting and Clinical Psychology*, *62*(3), 645–650. https://doi.org/10.1037/0022-006X.62.3.645

Quesenberry, A. C., Hemmeter, M. L., Ostrosky, M. M., & Hamann, K. (2014). Child care teachers' perspectives on including children with challenging behavior in child care settings. *Infants & Young Children*, *27*(3), 241–258. https://doi.org/10.1097/IYC.0000000000000012.

Reinke, W. M., Stormont, M., Herman, K. C., Puri, R., & Goel, N. (2011). Supporting children's mental health in schools: Teacher perceptions of needs, roles, and barriers. *School Psychology Quarterly*, *26*(1), 1–13. https://doi.org/10.1037/a0022714

Rosenzweig, J. M., Brennan, E. M., Huffstutter, K. J., & Bradley, J. R. (2008). Child care and employed parents of children with emotional or behavioral disorders. *Journal of Emotional and Behavioral Disorders*, *16*(2), 78–89. https://doi.org/10.1177/1063426607312538

Rosenzweig, J. M., Brennan, E. M., & Ogilvie, A. (2002). Work-family fit: Voices of parents of children with emotional and behavioral disorders. *Social Work*, *47*, 415–424. https://doi.org/10.1093/sw/47.4.415.

Sanchez, A. L., Cornacchio, D., Poznanski, B., Golik, A. M., Chou, T., & Comer, J. S. (2018). The effectiveness of school-based mental health services for elementary-aged children: A meta-analysis. *Journal of the American Academy of Child and Adolescent Psychiatry*, *57*(3), 153–165. https://doi.org/10.1016/j.jaac.2017.11.022

Sellmaier, C., & Buckingham, S. (2022). "I think sometimes that dads are kind of forgotten (…) so it's nice that we also get a voice.": Work-life experiences of employed U.S. fathers caring for a child with special health care needs. *Community, Work, & Family*, *25*(5), 661–676. https://doi.org/10.1080/13668803.2021.1911935

Sellmaier, C. (2019). Integrating work and family responsibilities: Experiences of fathers of children with special health care needs. *Journal of Child and Family Studies*, *28*(11), 3022–3036. https://doi.org/10.1007/s10826-019-01478-6

Sellmaier, C. (2021). Physical and mental health of mothers and fathers caring for children with special health care needs: The influence of community resources. *Journal of Family Issues*, *43*(11), 2815–2840. https://doi.org/10.1177/0192513X211035580

Sellmaier, C., Stewart, L. M., & Brennan, E. M. (2020). Workforce engagement of parents of children and youth with mental health difficulties: The impact of community services and supports. *Community Work & Family*, *23*(5), 534–555. https://doi.org/10.1080/13668803.2020.1820954

Shalaby, R. A. H., & Agyapong, V. I. O. (2022). Peer support in mental health: Literature review. *JMIR Ment Health*, *7*(6), e15572. https://doi.org/10.2196/15572

Sharko, M., Jameson, R., Ancker, J. S., Krams, L., Webber, E. C., & Rosenbloom, S. T. (2022). State-by-state variability in adolescent privacy laws. *Pediatrics*, *149* (6). https://doi.org/peds.2021-053458

Shilling, V., Morris, C., Thompson-Coon, J., Ukoumunne, O., Rogers, M., & Logan, S. (2013). Peer support for parents of children with chronic disabling conditions: A systematic review of quantitative and qualitative studies. *Developmental Medicine and Child Neurology*, *55*, 602–609. https://doi.org/10.1111/dmcn.12091

Tomopoulos, S., & Greenblatt, J. (2024). Integrated behavioral health care as a means of addressing common behavioral health concerns within pediatric primary care. *Current Problems in Pediatric and Adolescent Health Care*, *54*, 101715. https://doi.org/10.1016/j.cppeds.2024.101715

Tulli, M., Salami, B., Begashaw, L., Meherali, S., Yohani, S., & Hegadoren, K. (2020). Immigrant mothers' perspectives of barriers and facilitators in accessing mental health care for their children. *Journal of Transcultural Nursing*, *31*(6), 598–605. https://doi.org/10.1177/1043659620902812

U.S. Department of Education (n.d.). Individuals with Disabilities Education Act. Retrieved from: https://sites.ed.gov/idea/topic-areas/#LRE

U.S. Department of Education (2025). Section 504. Retrieved from: https://www.ed.gov/laws-and-policy/individuals-disabilities/section-504

U.S. Department of Justice Civil Rights Division (n.d.). Equal access to child care. Retrieved from: https://www.ada.gov/topics/child-care-centers/

Woolcock, S. C., Andrilla, C. H. A., Garberson, L. A., & Graves, J. M. (2025a) The supply and rural-urban distribution of the behavioral health workforce in Illinois. *Data Brief. WWAMI Rural Health Research Center*, University of Washington. Retrieved from: https://familymedicine.uw.edu/rhrc/wp-content/uploads/sites/4/2025/07/RHRC_DB-JUL2025_IL_BH_Woolcock.pdf

Woolcock, S. C., Andrilla, C. H. A., Garberson, L. A., & Graves, J. M. (2025b) The supply and rural-urban distribution of the behavioral health workforce in Washington. *Data Brief. WWAMI Rural Health Research Center*, University of Washington. Retrieved from: https://familymedicine.uw.edu/rhrc/wp-content/uploads/sites/4/2025/08/RHRC_DBAUG2025_WA_BH_Woolcock.pdf

7

THE EFFECTS OF COVID-19

This chapter will focus on the impact of the COVID-19 pandemic on work, family, and community systems. We will first examine the more immediate impacts in 2020 during the various forms of more extensive shutdowns discussing how these affected families and their exceptional care experiences. We will also look at any long-term and lingering effects that still shape work, family, and community systems. For example, telehealth or online mental health care remains a wide-spread option, possibly expanding access to care, while many employers greatly limit remote work options again, at times going even further than before the pandemic. The pandemic therefore casts a long shadow, shaping systems and services today, in addition to serving as a case study providing examples of possible changes that can have a positive impact on families with exceptional care responsibilities.

Part 1: Changes in Work and Community Systems, and Policy

Changes to Work

> I have needed to start working longer hours in my business to try and help my business survive. Meanwhile my husband has been furloughed.
>
> I work from home now, which is very difficult to do when I have a toddler at home who can't just be plopped into a playpen as a boss suggested. With one supervisor I have gone from being an extremely valued employee to an "unreliable employee because of the baby and his appointments".

The changes in the workplace during the immediate shutdown across the U.S. and in other countries played out in a variety of different ways for families. People in office jobs or professional roles usually moved to remote work, so-called front-line

DOI: 10.4324/9781003532668-7

workers including nurses, doctors, first-responders, or grocery workers kept going to their jobs dealing with the daily risk of exposure and quarantine requirements. Employees in the service industry working in restaurants or hotels might have lost their jobs altogether. The effects were therefore quite varied depending on the type of job and industry and the size of the employer.

According to the U.S. Census Bureau's American Community Survey, the rate of people working remotely increased from 5.7% in 2019 to 17.9% in 2021 (U.S. Census Bureau, 2022) and full-time employment declined by 4.4 million individuals (U.S. Census Bureau, 2022) resulting in a rise of the unemployment rate to 14.7% in April of 2020 (Bick & Blandin, 2020). The unemployment rate increased most sharply for low-income households with 28% reporting at least some time of the year being unemployed in 2020, compared to 14% of middle-income households and 8% of upper-income households (Kochar & Sechopoulos, 2022). Research also found some discrepancies in unemployment rates and job recovery for men and women (Hegewisch et al., 2025). The unemployment rate for women in April 2020 was 15.5%, while men's unemployment rate was 13%. By 2025, women's employment rates were back to pre-pandemic levels with a recovery time of three years, while men's employment rates recovered in closer to two years. Recovery was also slower for Black and Latina women who reported higher unemployment rates in September 2020, while the overall unemployment rate had already dropped to 7.9%, Black and Latina women remained at 11% (Ewing-Nelson, 2020). Unemployment was also higher for mothers than for fathers and especially pronounced for mothers with less than a bachelor's degree (Landivar, 2023). Employment of mothers with less than a bachelor's degree dropped by 22.1% and of mothers with a bachelor's degree or higher by 9.6% compared to fathers with less than a bachelor's degree dropping by 12.9% and fathers with a bachelor's degree or higher by 5.2%. Recovery for mothers with a bachelor's degree or less also had the slowest recovery reaching almost pre-pandemic levels with an employment rate of 98.9% by February 2023, while fathers of any level of education and mothers with a bachelor's degree or higher reached pre-pandemic levels closer toward the middle to end of 2022 and mothers with bachelor's degrees or higher and fathers with less than a bachelor's degree even surpassing pre-pandemic level employment rates by February 2023 (Landivar, 2023).

The U.S. Department of Homeland Security published an advisory list of essential workers defining these jobs as essential for the functioning of communities including safety, health, and economic and national security. In addition, several states developed their own guidelines for defining essential workers, making estimates of the actual number of essential workers difficult. Based on the number of people employed in 2018 in the industries identified by the Department of Homeland Security, the number could have ranged from 49 to 62 million people (Tomer & Kane, 2020) or up to 70% of all workers (Blau et al., 2021). If only considering workers who had to work face-to-face, the number might have been lower around 43% and when considering the effects of the shutdown only about 34% of essential frontline workers might have engaged in face-to-face work (Blau et al., 2021). Independent of the differences in the estimates of the total number of essential workers during the pandemic, research seems to agree that a majority of these frontline workers compared to all workers in the United States. were less educated, more likely to be immigrants, and earned lower average wages (Blau et al., 202; Geary et al., 2020; Monte & Laughlin, 2022).

Changes to Income and Benefits

The impact of these job changes on the economic situation of American households is also complicated and nuanced. All American households appeared to have lost income after inflation according to a Pew Research Center study (Kochar & Sechopoulos, 2022), but the losses were not equally distributed. For example, upper income households only reported .5% losses of annual income compared to 2% for middle income households and 3% for lower income households. This aligns with unemployment which hit lower-income households the hardest. Some households also reported changes in income tier from 2020 to 2021, with 32% of upper-income households dropping to middle-income households and 16% of middle-income households dropping to low-income households. This Pew study defined upper-income households as earning $180,020 annually for a family of four, and middle-income households earning $60,007. The study also found positive improvements with 32% of low-income households moving to the middle-income tier and 16% of middle-income households to the upper-income tier (Kochar & Sechopoulos, 2022). Federal and state governments approved changes to unemployment insurance, and the federal government passed several relief packages, such as the Families First Coronavirus Response Act and the Cares Act, which had a positive impact on overall household income. Interestingly, only 13% of low-income households reported receiving unemployment benefits despite an unemployment rate of 28%. Receipt of unemployment benefits was higher in middle- and upper-income households with 18% and 13% respectively (Kochar & Sechopoulos, 2022).

> Husband lost his job and we are paying high insurance premiums through COBRA. It is also affecting his ability to find a new job. This has added a great deal of stress to our relationship.

In addition to wage loss due to changes in employment, households potentially also faced the loss of health insurance, since health insurance in the United States is most often tied to employment. As mentioned in previous chapters, U.S. families have three main sources of health care insurance either through employment, private insurance either fully paid for by themselves or depending on their income subsidized by provisions of the Affordable Care Act or public insurance through Medicaid. Based on U.S. Census data one study found a 1.6% decline in employer-based health insurance from April to July 2020 and an increase of 1% in both uninsured and rate of individuals on public plans (Gangopadhyaya et al., 2020). The greatest loss of employer-based health insurance was reported by non-Hispanic Asian individuals with 7.6% followed by Hispanic individuals with 4.3%. Hispanic individuals also reported a significant increase in the uninsured rate with almost 4% reporting being uninsured. Decrease in employer-based health insurance was higher for individuals with a high school degree or less at 2.8% and an increase in individuals being uninsured by 1.6%. Changes in insurance status for individuals with some or more college education was minimal with 1% reporting losing employer-based insurance and .6% reporting no insurance at all. Not surprising, states who did not opt to expand Medicaid saw a greater increase in the number of individuals without health insurance than states who expanded Medicaid access (1.7% and .6%, respectively; Gangopadhyaya et al., 2020). The COVID-19 pandemic and its associated shutdowns therefore affected individuals and families in a variety of ways with some losing employment, some shifting to remote work, and some continuing face-to-face employment often with an increased risk to their own health. These changes, especially, the loss of employment, resulted in reductions of household income and possible loss of health insurance.

Changes to Services

> We are unable to schedule work commitments around school. In addition - we are not able to use friends/family to assist as needed.
>
> My son has not received any of his services outlined on his IEP. It has all fallen on my shoulders.

Changes to community services and systems were profound during the COVID-19 pandemic and the associated shutdowns. For example, all states in the United States had partial school closures starting in March of 2020 and all but two states kept schools closed for the remainder of the 2019/2020 school year. Starting the 2020/2021 school year one study of 100 urban school districts reported that the majority started off with remote learning (76%), which shifted over the course of the first semester to increasingly hybrid and in-person instruction with only 29% of school districts reporting fully remote instruction in February 2021 (Dusseault & Sharma, 2020) and four states requiring in-person instruction at the start of the 2020/2021 school year (Ferren, 2021). How remote instruction was implemented varied across school districts as well. For example, by the end of April 2020 only 44% of school districts provided a formal curriculum including instruction and progress monitoring, while 41% provided the curriculum without instruction or assessment (Lake & Dusseault, 2020). In the beginning at least, some schools provided paper packages for students to work through independently, others offered synchronous online instruction or a combination of both. Access to technology was addressed by many school districts at the beginning of the 2020/2021 school year according to experimental data, with 96% providing digital devices and 70%

at home internet access (National Center for Education Statistics, n.d.). Closure of child care was not as extensive as closure of K-12 education, but still widespread. According to data tracking, 15 states had specific mandates for child care closures mostly starting at the end of March 2020 until June at the latest (CUSP, n.d.). Another study found that 75% of child care centers closed in April 2020 and 25% remained closed one year later (Lee & Parolin, 2021). This study considered a child care center closed if it operated at less than 50% capacity. They also found that Black, Asian, and Latino families experienced child care closures at a greater rate than White families. The U.S. Department of Health and Human Services reported that 96% of Head Start early education centers were closed in April 2020 (Winston, 2021). These closures are especially impactful for low-income families and families caring for a child with a disability. For more information on these programs, please check Chapter 6. Based on a survey administered by the National Institute for Early Education Research, about 48% of preschool children received learning support while their programs were closed (Barnett et al., 2020).

> The pandemic has decreased already hard to find services. In addition, I currently have no respite or break.
>
> Neither child is able to be successful with virtual learning. The social isolation for child one ramped up all her issues and she ended up hospitalized for two weeks inpatient and an additional 5 weeks at partial hospitalization.

As mentioned above, health insurance coverage might have been disrupted for some families, impacting access to mental health care. Furthermore, stay-at-home orders resulted in the initial closure of outpatient mental health care

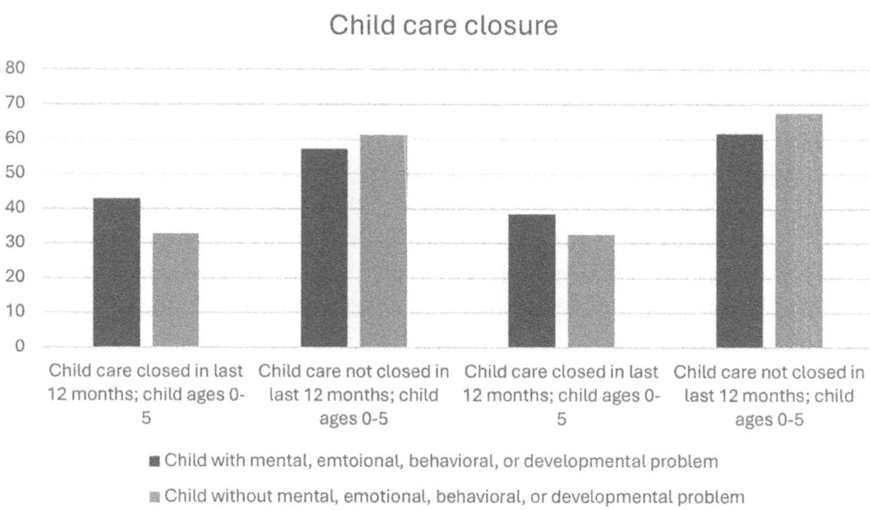

FIGURE 7.1 Child Care Closure Based on National Survey of Children's Health 2021

and the transition to telehealth or online mental health care. A survey conducted by the World Health Organization in August 2020 found disruptions to mental health service delivery across countries. For example, 72% of children and adolescents reported problems with their mental health services including disruptions to services delivered in schools, 30% shared changes to their medication access, and 35% experienced disruptions to the delivery of emergency services (World Health Organization, 2020). Restrictions to visitations also affected mental health hospitals and residential facilities, possibly limiting parent's ability to be with their children.

Federal Policy Changes

The COVID-19 pandemic also prompted federal legislation aimed at supporting individuals and families during this time of crisis. The two major policies we would like to briefly mention here are the Families First Coronavirus Response Act (FFCRA) and the Coronavirus Aid, Relief, and Economic Security Act (CARES Act). In the context of work provisions for paid Family and Medical Leave and sick leave are most critical for families. As discussed in earlier chapters, federal law in the United States only offers unpaid family and medical leave of up to 12 weeks for employees who have worked for at least one year at their job. The FFCRA (2020) enacted paid leave after the first ten days of unpaid leave for employees with at least 30 days on the job. Employees should receive two-thirds of their regular pay up to $200/day or $10,000 in total. The legislature added closure of schools and child care and the need to provide care as a reason to apply for leave. This act also entitled all employees to paid sick leave if they either contracted COVID-19, had to quarantine, or care for a child due to school and child care closures or other precautionary measures that required care. A full-time employee was eligible for up to 80 days of paid sick leave. The CARES Act also included direct relief payments to individuals and families. Individuals with an annual income below $75,000 and couples with less than $150,000 received $1,200 per adult and $500 per child. Households with incomes above this threshold received adjusted payments. The Tax Relief Act and the American Rescue Plan Act included provisions for additional direct payments to qualifying households in December 2020 and March 2021 (U.S. Department of the Treasury, n.d.). Pandemic Unemployment Assistance expanded access to unemployment benefits for individuals who either already exhausted their benefits or individuals who are usually not eligible for example, self-employed workers or workers with not enough time on a job. It also included a $600 weekly supplement to bolster the overall amount received by individuals and families (Center on Budget and Policy Priorities, 2021). The expansion of the child tax credit from $2,000 to $3,600, which was provided in full to all households including low-income households was another measure offering economic support to families (U.S. Department of the Treasury, n.d.).

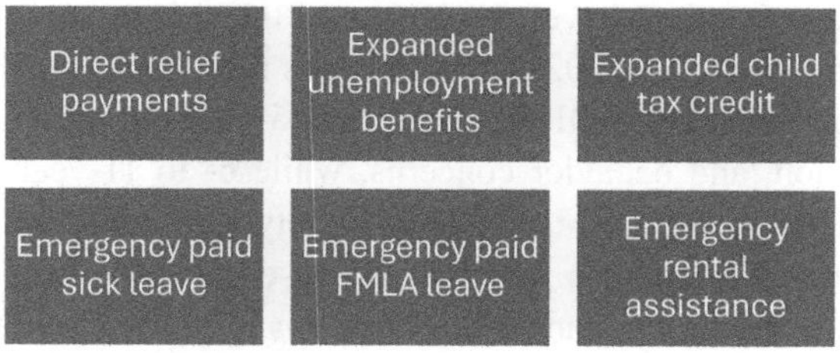

FIGURE 7.2 Pandemic Policies

Part 2: How These Changes Affected Families

> We had searched for the right therapist for years who could do trauma-informed work in American Sign Language, so we don't really know of an alternative. My son absolutely cannot connect with people on Zoom, so his relationships with his therapist and therapeutic mentor are both hanging on by a thread right.

> To be honest, not having to commute has made our days more relaxed. We have been hiking/getting out in nature since I can attend meetings via zoom.

> THEN the pandemic shut everything down and honestly, it was just the reset my daughter needed. And she's doing fine with the online schooling - at 13 and an introvert, it's a good transition for her.

The effects of these changes on the family system were manifold. For example, we conducted a survey study with families during the COVID-19 pandemic (Sellmaier & Kim, 2023) and parents shared that therapeutic services either fell away completely, especially if they were provided through schools, or were moved to telehealth settings. Remote services only worked for some children or did not work as well as in person services. The age of the child and types of symptoms seemed to play a role in how well online mental health care worked. For example, younger children might have responded less well and children with ADHD diagnosis might have had a harder time sitting still in front of a screen, especially if they already had to spend a few hours on a computer for school. Parents also shared that the mental health of their children deteriorated due to social isolation, less structure in their day, or the lack of physical activity since sports programs were canceled. One parent in our study said that their child had a mental health crisis and needed to be hospitalized, and they could not visit them during their stay. A systematic review confirms these findings stating that the mental health of children deteriorated during the COVID-19 pandemic (Ng & Ng, 2022; United Nations, 2020), which was also found in a U.K. survey among young people (YoungMinds, 2020). In this survey, young people identified the concerns about the pandemic and their schooling, the social isolation, the loss of structure and routine, and the loss or changes to existing mental health care as some factors contributing to their lower mental wellbeing. A

COVID-19 diagnosis might have also increased the risk for developing a mental health condition (West et al., 2021). Anxiety was most likely for 12–17-year-olds followed by depression and ADHD. Children 0–5-year-old most likely dealt with ADHD, depression, and behavior concerns, while 6- to 11-year-olds were most likely to experience symptoms of ADHD, anxiety, and adjustment disorder. The Center for Disease Control also found an increase in mental health-related emergency room visits during the pandemic (Leeb et al., 2020). Online schooling was a challenge as well and often required a lot of parental support. Families lost child care and respite care and were forced to spend a lot of time together, which also impacted the mental health of children and parents. Some lost their jobs due to the shutdowns, and others had to reduce hours or quit to meet the care demands at home, which affected income and increased financial worries. Trying to work from home and to manage children's educational needs was a great stressor and at times impossible (Sellmaier & Kim, 2023).

> My husband now works from home, which has actually helped. Now I can take the kids to medical appointments without worrying about childcare.

But the challenges do not make up the full picture of families' experiences during the pandemic and its associated shutdowns (Sellmaier & Kim, 2023). For example, parents shared that with both working from home, they were better able to share care responsibilities. They also appreciated spending less time in the car commuting to work or driving kids to various appointments and having more time to spend with family. Online therapeutic care worked well for some children and winning back time that was spent going to and from appointments was appreciated. Online schooling was also a positive experience for some families, who felt that they had more flexibility to structure the day, which helped children to deal better with the pressures of schoolwork. Parents whose children had struggled with relationships and social anxieties in school felt that their children were doing better away from the school setting. Some young people in the U.K. YoungMinds survey also shared that their mental health improved because they were not at school, which had been a place of stress or because they felt their own struggle with anxiety was now better understood and acknowledged by others (YoungMinds, 2020).

BOX 7.1 CASE SCENARIO

Ramona is a single mother of twin boys both of whom have been diagnosed with ADHD one month before the pandemic-related shutdowns. They both struggled in preschool, which prompted Ramona's visit to their pediatrician. Ramona found a therapist to start behavior training, but the shutdown stopped the therapy after a few visits. The boys' preschool closed, and they both struggled with the loss of routine showing more challenging behaviors than before. It is difficult to find opportunities for them to move around and release their energy since the local YMCA is closed, which they visit regularly to play in the pool or in the adventure zone. This was also always a great opportunity for Ramona to get a workout in while the boys were in the kids' zone, helping her deal with her stress. Ramona is a hair dresser and owns her own salon with two employees. She had to close the store and is glad that she received unemployment and rental assistance to make ends meet. She also received the first direct relief payment from the government, which was very helpful, but Ramona is stressed about how to keep paying the bills and buying groceries if she cannot open up her salon soon. Ramona's parents are elderly and live in another state and cannot help with child care. Ramona is also worried about their health and wishes she could help them with grocery shopping and errands so that they don't have to leave the house.

Governmental economic support programs and tax relief programs also had a positive impact on poverty rates. Based on U.S. Census Bureau data poverty rates dropped by 1.4% from 2020 to 2021 resulting in an overall 7.8% poverty rate (Creamer et al., 2022). Poverty rates declined most sharply for single female-headed households with a reduction of 6.4%, followed by children up to 18 years with a reduction of 4.5% and Black (3.3%) and Hispanic (2.8%) households, even though poverty remained higher for these households when compared to non-Hispanic white households with an overall poverty rate of 5.7%. An analysis by the Center on Budget Policy and Priorities (2023) showed that these drops in poverty were due to the governmental assistance programs and tax cuts. Accounting for these policy interventions, childhood poverty rates declined to 5.2%, while without government interventions, it was predicted that it would have been at 21.8% in 2021. These estimates included not just pandemic-related interventions, but previously established programs such as Supplemental Nutrition Assistance Program or the Earned Income Tax Credit.

Part 3: Trends Now and Long-term Effects

> My job ordered us all back to the office, due to my son's medical issues I was forced to take a leave of absence to be able to stay home. We have hired a nanny to care for the kids in our home. I had to find a different job so I could work remote.

One aspect of pandemic workplace changes was the option to work remotely. According to reporting from the Wall Street Journal (Williams, 2024), there has been a reduction in employees who work fully remotely and 16% of employees have mandates to work in the office five days/week. There is an increasing share of employees who are required to work at least some days in the office increasing from 63% in 2023 to 75% in 2024 (Parker, 2025). At the same time, hybrid schedules appeared to increase at the end of 2024 with 43% of employees reporting hybrid schedules compared to 29% one year prior. A schedule is considered hybrid if employees can at least work one day from home. Current trends as of the end of 2025 appear to be pointing toward continued efforts by companies to reduce remote work options. Some companies might have also used back-to-work requirements to reduce their workforce without laying anyone off. Employees remaining in remote work arrangements might get paid less than their in-office counterparts or might miss out on promotional opportunities. Overall, remote or hybrid schedules have remained a feature of the work environment, but there has also been backlash with big companies requiring employees to return to in-person work. It is also important to keep in mind that these types of place and time flexibility is only available to some types of jobs and are therefore only a support for some families. For example, only between 3% and 6% of employees working in the service industry, construction, transportation, or production reported some workplace flexibility compared to 36% in management or professional occupations (Richter, 2025). Paid leave policies therefore remain necessary to support employees in managing both workplace and family demands, especially for families with exceptional care demands who might encounter emergencies and crises more frequently. Even with remote work options being rolled back, I remain hopeful that the pandemic experience has opened the conversation. For example, even with an increase in back-to-work mandates, there are still 84% of employees who have some schedule flexibility, which is an increase from before the pandemic. Federal mandates for paid sick leave and paid FMLA expired in 2021, but there has been an increase in the number of states who have passed paid sick day laws. As of September 2025, there were 18 states with paid sick leave policies, an increase from 11 states before the pandemic (National Partnership for Women and Families, 2025). Employees in service industries, part-time workers, and workers in smaller companies are less likely to have access to paid sick leave. Only 39% of workers in the bottom 10% of income have access to paid leave compared to 96% in the top 10% of income, but low-income workers saw the greatest gain in access to sick leave from 2010 to 2023, from 20% to 39% (Gould & Wethin, 2023). There are also four additional states who passed paid FMLA laws since the pandemic and the U.S. House of Representatives passed a bill in 2021, which included paid FMLA leave. Unfortunately, the bill did not pass the Senate (Shabo, 2025). There might also be greater awareness and understanding of how difficult it can be to manage both work and care demands, since all families had to deal with this balancing act when schools and child care centers closed.

As discussed above, the federal government passed several financial programs to support families during the pandemic and its shutdowns. Unfortunately, similar to paid sick leave requirements, extensions to the Child Tax Credit were not passed beyond 2021. The impact of COVID-specific relief for families can be estimated when looking at the increase in poverty in 2022 once programs such as the extension of the Child Tax Credit expired. Childhood poverty rates increased again from 5.2% in 2021 to 12.4% in 2022 (Shrider & Creamer, 2023). Overall poverty rates also climbed to 12.4% surpassing the 2020 rate of 9.2%. Female-headed households, American Indian and Alaska Native households and individuals without a high school diploma were hit the hardest, seeing increases up to 11%. These are disturbing trends, and they also highlight the importance and effectiveness of government programs. The relief packages were successful in lowering the financial impact of the economic crisis. We can use this information as we continue to advocate for a more robust social safety net.

According to a 2025 Gallup poll, 21% of surveyed parents thought that the negative impact of the pandemic on their children's mental health persisted, and 22% thought that their children's social skill development was still affected (Brenan, 2025). The Youth Risk Behavior Survey found that 39.7% of high school students reported feeling sad or hopeless, which is a decrease from 42.3% in 2022, but still higher than in 2019 with 36.7% (Center for Disease Control, n.d.). LGBTQ+ and transgender students reported even higher levels with 65% of LGBTQ+ and 71% of transgender students reporting feeling sad or hopeless in 2023. Rates of suicide attempts also remained elevated in 2023 at 9.5% (Center for Disease Control, n.d.). The lasting impact on academic skills were rated slightly lower with 19% citing long-term effects on math, 16% on reading, and 14% on science. Parents whose children were in middle school during the pandemic were most likely to cite concerns, with 31% being concerned about mental health and social skills development. According to the National Assessment of Educational Progress NAEP's long term trends reports both reading and math scores for 9-year and for 13-year-olds were still lower in 2023 compared to 2020 assessments (National Assessment of Educational Progress, n.d.). School absenteeism increased after the pandemic-related school closures from 15% in 2018 to 28% in 2022 and remained high with 26% in 2023 (Rapaport et al., 2024). Academic performance, school attendance and mental wellbeing appear to be interconnected with students struggling in school and reporting more absences also being more likely to deal with mental health issues (Rapaport et al., 2024). These are correlations, and we cannot say if students who struggle with their mental health miss school or if missing school affects mental health or if both affect each other at the same time. Either way, it seems safe to argue that investments into mental health supports can boost academic success and mental health supports in schools can be considered a part of the academic work of the education system. Unfortunately, only 37% of low-income families and 29% of Black families reported that they had access to school-based mental health services compared to 59% of higher-income families and 52% of white families (Rapaport et al., 2024). This is especially problematic since low-income families who had access to school-based services were 5-times more likely to use them than higher-income families (55.5% compared to 10.8%, respectively). Considering the barriers to mental health care access discussed in Chapter 6, school-based services are also critical for parents to maintain employment, since they might not have the flexibility to drive their children to community-based services usually offered during regular work hours. Considering the trends in mental well-being since the pandemic and considering that many of the workplace and economic supports provided during the pandemic have been discontinued since then, makes the issues discussed in this book even more relevant today.

Part 4: Summary and Key Points

The pandemic and its associated shutdowns impacted families' economic situation and workplace conditions. They also affected children's child care and schooling situations, with services including mental health care falling away and with families trying to manage both work and care responsibilities often without outside support. These changes created additional stressors for both children and parents, and the effects are still felt today, when looking at the mental health of children and young adults and students' educational outcomes. The pandemic also led to emergency legislation such as federal paid sick leave and expansions of the child tax credit and increased workplace flexibility. Despite these changes being rolled back, they signal that change is possible and that effective social policies and workplace supports are critical and effective.

- Lasting changes to mental health service delivery with increased online care
- Potential effectiveness of social policies such as paid leave and child tax credits

Part 5: Implications for Social Work Practice

From a legislative perspective, social workers should continue to advocate for the expansion of the child tax credit including the provision that all families independent of income receive the full credit. Social work advocacy should also focus on federal paid sick leave and paid FMLA leave provisions for all employees. Data from the pandemic can bolster arguments for the effectiveness of these legislative interventions.

Online mental health care has been experienced as beneficial by some families. For example, scheduling was easier, since parents did not have to budget time for travel. Families living in areas with fewer providers also have access to a larger network if care can be accessed remotely. Online care also requires access to technology, internet, and a private space, which can be an access barrier. Online care might be less effective for younger children or children with specific diagnoses or co-occurring disorders. Social work research should therefore continue to examine the effectiveness of remote care for children of different ages and across different diagnoses. Social work programs should train their students in providing effective remote services since remote care will remain a consistent aspect of mental health service provisions. The question also remains how mental health care can be provided with greater flexibility and access, since online mental health care won't work for everyone. Increasing mental health care in school settings could be one tool to achieve this goal.

Part 6: Application for Social Work Education

ACTIVITY 1: DISCUSSION QUESTIONS

- How did the COVID-19 pandemic affect you, your friends, and family?
- Do you notice any lingering, long-term effects?
- How might your experience be the same or different from the information you read in this chapter?
- What are some of the unique challenges families caring for a child with a mental health disability faced?
- What lessons can we learn to improve social services and social policies today?

ACTIVITY 2: WORKING WITH A FAMILY DURING THE PANDEMIC

Competency 6: Engage with Individuals, Families, Groups, Organizations, and Communities
Competency 7: Assess Individuals, Families, Groups, Organizations, and Communities
Competency 8: Intervene with Individuals, Families, Groups, Organizations, and Communities

Examine the case study from Chapter 4 and discuss how the family might have fared during the pandemic.

Pre-pandemic situation: Julia (mother, 42), Robert (father, 47), Maria (daughter, 12), and Ben (son, 10) Hunter just moved to a new state, because Robert was offered a better-paying position at a non-profit agency. Julia is currently looking for a new position as an accountant. Money is tighter right now, since Julia is not working. Maria and Ben are both enrolled in public schools, Maria in a large middle school and Ben in a small elementary school. Maria has recently been diagnosed with depression and an eating disorder, which upended the family's routines. Maria participates in an outpatient half-day treatment program. Julia is driving Maria to the clinic at 8am in the morning and picks her up at 1pm. Robert is helping Ben in the mornings and makes sure he gets on the school bus before heading to work. Maria is not going to school right now and has to be supervised. Maria and Julia spend the afternoon together until they pick up Ben from school. Robert often comes home late from work, since he is still learning his new job. Luckily, Robert's job comes with good health insurance and the out-of-pocket payments for Maria's current treatment is manageable. The family doesn't have friends yet, since they just moved to the new town. Julia and Robert left behind their parents and siblings. While they don't have any family members in the area, they all feel very connected to each other. Ben has been acting out at home and at school. His school has called his parents for a meeting, since Ben hit another schoolmate in a fight over the monkey bars. You are a social worker in Maria's clinic, and you work with the family members of the children receiving treatment.

- How would the pandemic affect the family's employment and economic situation?
- How would it affect their access to schooling and mental health care?
- How could the pandemic affect the mental health of all family members and the family relationships?
- How would you as the social worker of the treatment facility support the family during the pandemic?

ACTIVITY 3: POLICY ADVOCACY AND ANALYSIS

Competency 2: Advance Human Rights and Social, Racial, Economic, and Environmental Justice
Competency 5: Engage in Policy Practice

The pandemic and the emergency policies passed during the pandemic can be used as a case study for policy advocacy. Students can research the policies and their impact on families such as family Hunter, using a policy analysis framework. Resources below can help with the research. The following questions can inform the policy analysis:

- What benefit/service is provided by the program?
- Who is eligible for the benefit?
- Does it reach the intended population, especially when considering the needs of children with mental health disabilities?
- Is everyone covered adequately, especially when considering mental health needs?

Since most of these emergency legislations have expired, students can use the collected information to develop an advocacy plan. For example, they could send a letter to their legislator, or write an editorial to their newspaper, sharing what they learned and why these policies would be beneficial.

Resource List

Brookings https://www.brookings.edu/
Center on Budget and Policy Priorities: https://www.cbpp.org/
Economic Policy Institute https://www.epi.org/
U.S. Department of Treasury: Covid-19 economic relief: https://home.treasury.gov/policy-issues/coronavirus

References

Barnett, S., Jung, K., & Milagros, N. (2020). Young children's home learning and preschool participation experiences during the pandemic. *NIEER 2020 Preschool Learning Activities Survey: Technical Report and Selected Findings*. Retrieved from: https://nieer.org/sites/default/files/2023-08/NIEER_Tech_Rpt_July2020_Young_Childrens_Home_Learning_and_Preschool_Participation_Experiences_During_the_Pandemic-AUG2020.pdf

Bick, A., & Blandin, A. (2020). Real time labor market estimates during the coronavirus outbreak. *W. P. Carey School of Business*.

Blau, F. D., Koebe, J., & Meyerhofer, P. A. (2021). Who are the essential and frontline workers? *Business Economics*, *56*(3), 168–178. https://doi.org/10.1057/s11369-021-00230-7.

Brenan, M. (2025). Pandemic hurt children's social skills, mental health most. *Gallup*. Retrieved from: https://news.gallup.com/poll/658100/pandemic-hurt-children-social-skills-mental-health.aspx

Center on Budget and Policy Priorities (2021). Policy basics: Unemployment insurance. Retrieved from: https://www.cbpp.org/research/economy/unemployment-insurance

Center on Budget Policy and Priorities (2023). Government's pandemic response turned a would-be poverty surge into a record poverty decline. Retrieved from: https://www.cbpp.org/research/poverty-and-inequality/governments-pandemic-response-turned-a-would-be-poverty-surge-into

Center on Budget Policy and Priorities (2024). Expiration of pandemic relief led to record increases in poverty and child poverty in 2022. Retrieved from: https://www.cbpp.org/research/poverty-and-inequality/expiration-of-pandemic-relief-led-to-record-increases-in-poverty

Centers for Disease Control and Prevention (CDC). 1991–2023 high school youth risk behavior survey data. Retrieved from: http://yrbs-explorer.services.cdc.gov/.

Creamer, J., Shrider, E. A., Burns, K., & Chen, F. (2022). Poverty in the United States: 2021. Current population reports. Retrieved from: https://www.census.gov/content/dam/Census/library/publications/2022/demo/p60-277.pdf

CUSP (n.d.). Covid-19 US state policies: Data library. *Boston University*. Retrieved from: https://statepolicies.com

Dusseault, B., & Sharma, R. (2020). Community health, vaccination policies & local preference: How 100 districts are reopening after COVID-19 shutdowns. Retrieved from: https://crpe.org/community-health-vaccination-policies-local-preference-how-100-districts-are-reopening-after-covid-19-shutdowns/

Ewing-Nelson, C. (2020). Four times more women than men dropped out of the labor force in September. *National Women's Law Center*. Retrieved from: https://nwlc.org/wp-content/uploads/2020/10/september-jobs-fs1.pdf

Families First Coronavirus Response Act (2020). Retrieved from: https://www.congress.gov/116/plaws/publ127/PLAW-116publ127.pdf

Ferren, M. (2021). Remote learning and school reopenings: What worked and what didn't. *Center for American Progress*. Retrieved from: https://www.americanprogress.org/article/remote-learning-school-reopenings-worked-didnt/

Gangopadhyaya, A., Karpman, M., & Aarons, J. (2020). As the COVID-19 recession extended into the summer of 2020, more than 3 million adults lost employer-sponsored health insurance coverage and 2 million became uninsured: Evidence from the Household Pulse Survey, April 23–July 21, 2020. *Urban Institute*. Retrieved from: https://www.urban.org/sites/default/files/publication/102852/as-the-covid-19-recession-extended-into-the-summer-of-2020-more-than-3-million-adults-lost-employer-sponsored-health-insurance-coverage-and-2-million-became-uninsured.pdf

Geary, C., Palacios, V., & Tatum, L. (2020). Who are essential workers. Retrieved from https://www.georgetownpoverty.org/wp-content/uploads/2020/07/GCPI-ESOI-Essential-Workers-July2020.pdf

Gould, E., & Wethin, H. (2023). Paid sick leave access expands with widespread state action: Low-wage workers without access face economic and health insecurity. *Economic Policy Institute.* Retrieved from: https://www.epi.org/publication/paid-sick-leave-2023/

Hegewisch, A., James, M. S., Mahoney, M., & Mendoza, C. (2025). Women at work five years since the start of the Covid-19 pandemic: Any progress? *Institute for Women's Policy Research.* Retrieved from: https://iwpr.org/wp-content/uploads/2025/03/Women-at-Work-Five-Years-Since-the-Start-of-the-COVID-19-Pandemic-fact-sheet_March-2025.pdf

Kochar, R., & Sechopoulos, S. (2022). COVID-19 pandemic pinches finances of America's lower- and middle-income families. *Pew Research Center.* Retrieved from: https://www.pewresearch.org/social-trends/2022/04/20/covid-19-pandemic-pinches-finances-of-americas-lower-and-middle-income-families/

Lake, R., & Dusseault, B. (2020). Remote classes are in session for more school districts, but attendance plans are still absent. Retrieved from: https://crpe.org/remote-classes-are-in-session-for-more-school-districts-but-attendance-plans-are-still-absent/

Landivar, C. (2023). Pandemic employment losses worse for working moms without degrees. *U.S. Department of Labor Blog.* Retrieved from: https://blog.dol.gov/2023/05/11/pandemic-employment-losses-worse-for-working-moms-without-degrees#:~:text=Following%20a%20significant%20decline%20in%20employment%20in,has%20not%20reached%20all%20groups%20of%20mothers.

Lee, E. K., & Parolin, Z. (2021). The care burden during COVID-19: A national database of child care closures in the United States. *Socius: Sociological Research for a Dynamic World, 7.* https://doi.org/10.1177/23780231211032028

Leeb, R. T., Bitsko, R. H., Radhakrishnan, L., Martinez, P., Njai, R., & Holland, K. M. (2020). Mental health-related emergency department visits among children aged <18 years during the COVID-19 pandemic—United States. *MMWR Morb Mortal Wkly Rep, 69*, 1675–1680. http://dx.doi.org/10.15585/mmwr.mm6945a3

Monte, L. M., & Laughlin, L. (2022). Essential, front-line and high-risk: How Covid-19 prioritized low-wage workers while heightening their disadvantage. *U.S. Census Bureau.* Retrieved from: https://www.census.gov/content/dam/Census/library/working-papers/2022/demo/sehsd-wp2022-08.pdf

National Assessment of Educational Progress (n.d.). Explore NAEP long term trends in reading and mathematics. Retrieved from: https://www.nationsreportcard.gov/ltt/?age=13

National Center for Education Statistics (n.d.). U.S. education in the time of Covid. Retrieved from: https://nces.ed.gov/surveys/annualreports/topical-studies/covid/?educationType=elementary-and-secondary-education

National Partnership for Women and Families (2025). Current paid sick days laws. Retrieved from: https://nationalpartnership.org/wp-content/uploads/2023/02/current-paid-sick-days-laws.pdf

Ng, C. S. M., & Ng, S. S. L. (2022). Impact of the COVID-19 pandemic on children's mental health: A systematic review. *Front Psychiatry, 18*(13), 975936. https://doi.org/10.3389/fpsyt.2022.975936.

Parker, K. (2025). Many remote workers say they'd be likely to leave their job if they could no longer work from home. *Pew Research Center.* Retrieved from: https://www.pewresearch.org/short-reads/2025/01/13/many-remote-workers-say-theyd-be-likely-to-leave-their-job-if-they-could-no-longer-work-from-home/

Rapaport, A., Polikoff, M., Saavedra, A., & Silver, D. (2024). A nation's children at risk: Insights on children's mental health from the Understanding America Study. University of Southern California. Retrieved from: http://uasdata.usc.edu/education

Richter, F. (2025). Which jobs are most often done remotely? *Statista.* Retrieved from: https://www.statista.com/chart/34444/share-of-remote-workers-by-occupation-group/

Sellmaier, C., & Kim, J. (2023). Working and caring for a disabled, adopted child during a pandemic. *Child and Family Social Work, 28*(1), 222–235. https://doi.org/10.1111/cfs.12955

Shabo, V. (2025). Explainer: Paid leave benefits and funding in the United States. *New America.* Retrieved from: https://www.newamerica.org/better-life-lab/briefs/explainer-paid-leave-benefits-and-funding-in-the-united-states/

Shrider, E. A., & Creamer, J. (2023). Poverty in the United States: 2022. Current population reports. Retrieved from: https://www.census.gov/content/dam/Census/library/publications/2023/demo/p60-280.pdf

Tomer, A., & Kane, J. W. (2020). How to protect essential workers during Covid-19. Retrieved from: https://www.brookings.edu/articles/how-to-protect-essential-workers-during-covid-19/

U.S. Census Bureau (2022). The number of people primarily working from home tripled between 2019 and 2021. Retrieved from: https://www.census.gov/newsroom/press-releases/2022/people-working-from-home.html

U.S. Department of the Treasury (n.d.). Assistance for American families and workers. Retrieved from: https://home.treasury.gov/policy-issues/coronavirus/assistance-for-American-families-and-workers

United Nations (2020). Policy brief: Covid 19 and the need for action on mental health. Retrieved from: https://www.un.org/sites/un2.un.org/files/un_policy_brief-covid_and_mental_health_final.pdf

West, K. D., Ali, M. M., Schreier, A., & Plourde, E. (2021). Child and adolescent mental health during COVID-19: Considerations for schools and early childhood providers (Issue Brief). Washington, DC: Office of the Assistant Secretary for Planning and Evaluation, U.S. Department of Health and Human Services. Retrieved from: https://aspe.hhs.gov/sites/default/files/documents/0bcc372f4755cca29ebc80a47cfe300e/child-adolescent-mh-covid.pdf

Williams, J. (2024). Will 2025 be the watershed year for return-to-office mandates? That Depends. *The Wall Street Journal*. Retrieved from: https://www.wsj.com/articles/will-2025-be-the-watershed-year-for-return-to-office-mandates-that-depends-11047d9a

Winston, P. (2021). COVID-19 and economic opportunity: Unequal effects on economic need and program response. *Office of the Assistant Secretary for Planning & Evaluation, U.S. Department of Health & Human Services.* Retrieved from: https://aspe.hhs.gov/sites/default/files/private/pdf/265391/covid-19-human-service-response-brief.pdf

World Health Organization (2020). COVID-19 disrupting mental health services in most countries. *WHO Survey.* Retrieved from: https://www.who.int/news/item/05-10-2020-covid-19-disrupting-mental-health-services-in-most-countries-who-survey

YoungMinds (2020). Coronavirus: Impact on young people with mental health needs. Retrieved from: https://www.youngminds.org.uk/media/xq2dnc0d/youngminds-coronavirus-report-march2020.pdf

8

COMPARATIVE ANALYSIS OF DEVELOPED COUNTRIES' POLICIES

This chapter examines how national social policy frameworks shape the experiences of families raising children with mental health disabilities, often under conditions of uncertainty as families navigate fragmented and evolving systems of support. Rather than approaching children's mental health primarily through clinical or educational systems, the analysis situates mental health disability within broader welfare arrangements that structure access to services, define eligibility, and distribute responsibility for care among the state, the market, and families.

Using a comparative policy approach informed by welfare regime theory, the chapter analyzes the United States, Canada, and Germany. Although the United States and Canada are typically classified as liberal welfare regimes, they differ in how health care, education, and income supports are organized and accessed. Germany represents a conservative-corporatist welfare regime in which social insurance plays a more central role, and caregiving is more formally recognized. Examining these cases highlights how policy design shapes not only family experiences, but also the forms of navigation, coordination, and advocacy that increasingly fall to social workers supporting children and their caregivers across systems.

Part 1: Comparative Policy Framework

This chapter combines welfare regime theory with a comparative policy mapping approach commonly used in cross-national family policy research. The analysis first identifies the statutory policy frameworks affecting families across domains including health care, education, income supports, caregiving leave, and anti-discrimination protections (Table 8.2). It then examines key policy design features that shape how these frameworks operate in practice (Table 8.3). Guided by a disability justice lens, we then center the analysis on how policy designs distribute care, risk, and responsibility

DOI: 10.4324/9781003532668-8

across families, markets, and the state, often reproducing ableist assumptions about caregiving, productivity, and deservingness. Access to support, caregiving burden, and exposure to financial and employment insecurity are thus understood not as consequences of diagnosis alone, but as outcomes of policy architectures that differentially value care and constrain families' ability to meet their children's needs.

Within welfare regime theory, liberal welfare states are characterized by greater reliance on market provision, means-tested programs, and employment-linked benefits, with public supports often operating as conditional or residual. Conservative-corporatist welfare states, by contrast, rely more heavily on social insurance and status-preserving benefits, with caregiving and disability more explicitly incorporated into statutory systems. These distinctions are analytically relevant for understanding children's mental health policy, as they influence how responsibility for care is distributed, whether caregiving labor is formally recognized, and the extent to which families absorb financial and coordination risks.

We selected three high-income countries to illustrate how countries with similar levels of economic and human development organize social protections in response to children's mental health needs. It is helpful to begin this analysis using comparative social indicators such as population size, gross domestic product (GDP), the Human Development Index (HDI), and the Gender Development Index (GDI). These indicators establish that the countries examined are all high-income economies with substantial fiscal capacity. Differences in policy responses to children's mental health disability therefore reflect *institutional design and political choice* rather than resource scarcity.

Table 8.2 summarizes the primary policy frameworks affecting families raising children with mental health disabilities across the United States, Canada, and Germany. The table brings together *key statutes and programs* across *four policy domains* that structure how families access support: *health care systems, education policies, financial supports and caregiving leave, and anti-discrimination protections*. Presenting these policies side by side provides an overview of the *institutional architecture* through which children's mental health needs are recognized and addressed within each country.

Across the three countries, mental health disability is addressed through multiple policy sectors rather than a single integrated system. Health care policies determine access to diagnostic assessment and treatment, education systems provide accommodations and school-based supports, financial supports and leave policies shape families' ability to sustain caregiving while maintaining employment, and anti-discrimination laws establish legal protections in workplaces and other institutional settings. Table 8.2 also highlights how these domains are governed by distinct statutory frameworks in each country, reflecting broader welfare regime arrangements that influence how responsibility for care is distributed among families, the state, and the market. By mapping these policy frameworks together, the table provides a foundation for the sector-specific analyses that follow in the subsequent sections of the chapter.

TABLE 8.1 Comparative Indicators for the United States, Germany, and Canada

Indicator	*United States*	*Germany*	*Canada*
Population (2024)	~340 million	~84 million	~41 million
Gross Domestic Product (GDP, current US$)	~$29.2 trillion	~$4.66 trillion	~$2.24 trillion
Human Development Index (HDI)	0.938	0.959	0.939
Gender Development Index (GDI)	1.009	0.975	0.991
Child and youth mental health prevalence	~20–28% of children aged 3–17 report a current mental or behavioral health condition	~22–28% of children and adolescents show signs of mental health problems	~15–20% of children and youth report a mental health condition

Notes

Population and GDP: Population size and GDP (current US$) are derived from World Bank Open Data (2024 estimates) for the United States, Germany, and Canada.

Human Development Index (HDI): HDI values are drawn from the United Nations Development Programme *Human Development Report 2023/2024* and reflect composite measures of life expectancy, education, and income.

Gender Development Index (GDI): GDI values are drawn from the United Nations Development Programme (latest available estimates). Values close to 1 indicate near gender parity in human development achievements.

Child and youth mental health prevalence: Prevalence estimates are derived from nationally representative population surveys and are not directly comparable across countries due to differences in age ranges, measurement instruments, and reporting methods.

United States: Parent-reported prevalence estimates from the National Survey of Children's Health (NSCH) indicate that approximately 20.3% of adolescents aged 12–17 had a diagnosed mental or behavioral health condition in 2023, with broader estimates of mental, behavioral, or developmental disorders (MBDDs) ranging from approximately 25–28% among children aged 3–17 (CDC; Maternal and Child Health Bureau).

Germany: Estimates are drawn from the BELLA study, the mental health module of the German Health Interview and Examination Survey for Children and Adolescents (KiGGS), which reports that approximately 21.9% of children and adolescents aged 7–17 show clinically relevant emotional or behavioral problems based on standardized screening instruments.

Canada: Estimates are derived from population surveys conducted by Statistics Canada. The last nationally representative diagnostic prevalence estimates for specific mental disorders were published in the Canadian Community Health Survey – Mental Health (2012). More recent data are reported as trend indicators from annual CCHS cycles (2015–2022) and screening-based measures from the Canadian Health Survey on Children and Youth, indicating that approximately 15–20% of children and youth report a mental health condition.

Our cross-national analysis also includes an assessment of policy design characteristics found in Table 8.3. Table 8.3 summarizes key policy design features affecting families raising children with mental health disabilities across the three countries. Policy dimensions reflect *structural characteristics* of health care systems, education supports, income protections, caregiving leave policies, and anti-discrimination

TABLE 8.2 Policy Frameworks Affecting Parents of Children with Mental Health Disabilities: United States, Canada, and Germany

Policy domain	*United States*	*Canada*	*Germany*
Health Care Coverage	Medicaid (including EPSDT), Children's Health Insurance Program (CHIP), Affordable Care Act (ACA) essential health benefits, Mental Health Parity and Addiction Equity Act (MHPAEA)	Public health insurance under the Canada Health Act, administered by provincial systems (e.g., Ontario Health Insurance Plan, Alberta Health Care Insurance Plan); provincial child and youth mental health programs; Integrated Youth Services models (e.g., Foundry BC)	Statutory Health Insurance (Gesetzliche Krankenversicherung – GKV); coverage for child and adolescent psychiatry and psychotherapy under the Social Code Book V (SGB V)
Disability Recognition/ Legal Definition	Americans with Disabilities Act (ADA); Section 504 of the Rehabilitation Act; Individuals with Disabilities Education Act (IDEA)	Canadian Human Rights Act and provincial human rights codes recognizing disability; federal disability framework through Accessible Canada Act	Social Code Book IX (SGB IX) defining disability and participation rights; implementation aligned with the UN Convention on the Rights of Persons with Disabilities (CRPD)
Education Supports	Individuals with Disabilities Education Act (IDEA) providing Individualized Education Programs (IEPs); Section 504 Plans under the Rehabilitation Act	Provincial education legislation and inclusive education policies (e.g., Education Act Ontario, School Act British Columbia); accommodation rights under provincial human rights codes	Inclusive education frameworks under state (Länder) education laws; supports through Schulbegleitung (school aides); Eudctaion ins separate Förderschulen still exist as well; participation supports under SGB VIII §35a
Income Supports for Families	Supplemental Security Income (SSI) for children with disabilities; Child Tax Credit; Medicaid eligibility linked to SSI in many states	Canada Child Benefit (CCB); Child Disability Benefit (CDB); Disability Tax Credit (DTC); some provincial disability programs	Kindergeld (Child Benefit); Pflegeversicherung (Long-Term Care Insurance) providing Pflegegeld cash benefits and in-kind services; disability participation supports under SGB IX

(*Continued*)

TABLE 8.2 (Continued)

Policy domain	*United States*	*Canada*	*Germany*
Caregiving Leave Policies	Family and Medical Leave Act (FMLA) (unpaid job-protected leave); state paid family leave programs in some states (e.g., California Paid Family Leave)	Employment Insurance Caregiving Benefits, including Parents of Critically Ill Children Benefit; job-protected family leave provisions in provincial employment standards legislation	Pflegezeitgesetz (Caregiver Leave Act); Familienpflegezeitgesetz (Family Caregiver Leave Act); Elterngeld/Elternzeit parental leave provisions
Employment Anti-Discrimination Protections	Americans with Disabilities Act (ADA) association discrimination protections; some state or local family responsibilities discrimination protections	Canadian Human Rights Act (federal) and provincial human rights codes protecting disability and family status; duty to accommodate caregiving responsibilities	Allgemeines Gleichbehandlungsgesetz (AGG) (General Equal Treatment Act); protections reinforced by European Court of Justice rulings recognizing discrimination against caregivers of disabled persons
Caregiving Supports in Social Insurance	None at federal level; support largely through means-tested programs	Limited direct caregiving allowance: support delivered through tax benefits and EI programs	Pflegeversicherung (Long-Term Care Insurance) providing graded cash and service benefits based on Pflegegrad assessments

TABLE 8.3 Policy Design Features Shaping Access to Services and Supports in the United States, Canada, and Germany

Policy dimension	*United States*	*Canada*	*Germany*
Health care coverage model	Mixed public–private insurance system combining employer-sponsored insurance, Medicaid, and CHIP	Universal publicly funded physician and hospital care under provincial health insurance systems	Universal statutory health insurance system (Gesetzliche Krankenversicherung)
Coverage of child mental health treatment	Covered through private insurance and Medicaid; mental health parity required under MHPAEA and ACA essential health benefits	Psychiatric care covered under public health insurance; psychotherapy and community services often outside public coverage	Child and adolescent psychiatry and psychotherapy covered within statutory insurance
Access to non-physician mental health services	Often dependent on insurance network and cost sharing	Frequently private pay or extended insurance unless delivered through publicly funded programs	Covered through statutory insurance but constrained by provider supply
School-based disability supports	Federal statutory rights under IDEA and Section 504; IEPs and accommodation plans required	Provincial inclusive education frameworks and accommodation duties under human rights law	Educational supports determined through state-level assessment systems and inclusion policies
Direct income support for families	Supplemental Security Income (SSI) for children with severe disabilities; strict means testing	Canada Child Benefit (CCB) and Child Disability Benefit (CDB) linked to Disability Tax Credit eligibility	Child benefit (Kindergeld) plus long-term care insurance benefits (Pflegegeld) for children with recognized care needs
Institutional recognition of caregiving	Limited recognition; caregiving support largely indirect	Partial recognition through tax benefits and EI caregiving programs	Explicit recognition through long-term care insurance and statutory caregiver supports
Caregiving leave availability	Federal job-protected leave under the Family and Medical Leave Act (FMLA); unpaid	Employment Insurance caregiving benefits for parents of critically ill children plus provincial job-protected leave	Statutory caregiving leave programs under Pflegezeitgesetz and Familienpflegezeitgesetz

(Continued)

TABLE 8.3 (Continued)

Policy dimension	*United States*	*Canada*	*Germany*
Wage replacement during caregiving leave	None at federal level (leave unpaid); some at individual state level	Partial wage replacement through Employment Insurance benefits	Partial income replacement or financial support depending on leave program
Eligibility constraints for leave	Employer size and employment tenure requirements	Eligibility linked to Employment Insurance contributions and labor force attachment	Employment and employer size thresholds for some leave provisions
Recognition of long-term caregiving needs	Limited policy recognition outside SSI eligibility	Partial recognition but benefits often designed for short-term care episodes	Stronger recognition through long-term care insurance and graded care levels
Employment discrimination protections	ADA protections against discrimination based on association with a person with a disability	Human rights legislation protecting disability and family status	Anti-discrimination protections under the General Equal Treatment Act (AGG)
System coordination and navigation burden	High fragmentation across health insurance, education systems, and social programs	Moderate to high coordination across provincial systems and programs	More standardized systems but still bureaucratic and assessment-based

Note: The table summarizes key policy design features affecting families raising children with mental health disabilities in the United States, Canada, and Germany. Policy dimensions reflect structural characteristics of health care systems, education supports, income protections, caregiving leave policies, and anti-discrimination protections. The comparison highlights how institutional design influences access to services, financial protection, and caregiving responsibilities across countries.

protections. The comparison highlights how *institutional design* influences variation in *access to services, financial protection, and caregiving responsibilities* across the three countries.

Defining Mental Health Disability in Children

A central premise of this chapter is that how governments define mental health disability determines who is recognized, who is eligible for support, and which families receive protection.

United States

In the United States, mental health disability is explicitly defined in federal law. Under the Americans with Disabilities Act, a disability includes mental impairments that substantially limit one or more major life activities (42 U.S.C. § 12102). For children, this definition is operationalized through Section 504 of the Rehabilitation Act and the Individuals with Disabilities Education Act (IDEA), which rely on functional impact on educational performance and the need for services rather than diagnosis alone (Individuals with Disabilities Education Act, 2004).

Canada

Canada does not have a single federal statutory definition of mental health disability specific to children. Disability is defined broadly as the interaction between physical, mental, or psychological impairments and environmental barriers that limit participation. Disabilities may be permanent, temporary, or episodic (Human Resources and Skills Development Canada [HRSDC], 2013). Mental health disabilities are recognized within federal and provincial human rights frameworks when mental impairments substantially limit functioning or participation (Ontario Human Rights Commission, 2014). Children are identified as having a disability for policy purposes when mental health or neurodevelopmental conditions significantly interfere with learning, emotional regulation, social interaction, or daily functioning, though eligibility varies across programs and provinces.

Germany

Germany defines disability through Book IX of the Social Code (SGB IX) as long-term physical, mental, intellectual, or psychological impairments that limit participation in society for more than six months. Mental health disabilities are explicitly included when psychological impairments interfere with age-appropriate functioning (Sozialgesetzbuch IX). This definition aligns with the UN Convention on the Rights of Persons with Disabilities, which Germany has ratified (United Nations, 2006).

Part 2: Health Care Coverage and Mental Health Policy Responses

Across the United States, Canada, and Germany, mental health disability is formally recognized when it substantially limits functioning or participation in daily life, including learning, social interaction, and emotional regulation. Despite this shared definitional foundation, the criteria used to establish eligibility, the processes through which needs are assessed, and the administrative consequences that follow vary considerably across countries. As the chapter turns to specific policy sectors, these differences become more apparent, as policy responses are shaped by distinct welfare regime logics that influence how responsibility for care is allocated, how risk is distributed between families and the state, and how supports are operationalized in practice. The purpose of this section is to document how health care systems are organized and accessed in each national context; comparative analysis of implications for families and social work practice is taken up later in the chapter. The following subsection describes the organization of children's mental health care within the U.S. health system, with attention to coverage, service pathways, and access mechanisms.

United States: Health Care and Mental Health Policy Responses

Mental health care for children in the United States is delivered through a highly fragmented, mixed public–private system. Access to services is shaped by insurance status, state policy decisions, and provider availability, resulting in substantial variation across families and regions. Children's mental health services are financed primarily through private insurance, Medicaid, and the Children's Health Insurance Program (CHIP), with eligibility and coverage differing significantly across states. Private insurance remains the dominant source of coverage for children, but access to mental health services depends on plan design, provider networks, and cost-sharing requirements. The Mental Health Parity and Addiction Equity Act (MHPAEA) requires parity between mental health and medical benefits in group health plans, and the Affordable Care Act (ACA) further designated mental health and substance use treatment as essential health benefits (Beronio et al., 2013). Despite these protections, families frequently encounter limited provider networks, high out-of-pocket costs, and long wait times for child and adolescent mental health specialists (Lynch & Dickerson, 2012; National Center for Health Workforce Analysis, 2024). Public coverage through Medicaid and CHIP plays a critical role for children with mental health disabilities, particularly those from low-income families. Medicaid is the largest payer of children's mental health services in the United States and is required to cover Early and Periodic Screening, Diagnostic, and Treatment (EPSDT) services, which mandate comprehensive and preventive health services for enrolled children. EPSDT theoretically offers robust coverage for mental health screening and treatment, but implementation varies widely across states, and service availability is often constrained by workforce shortages and administrative barriers (Peters, 2006). For children with significant mental health needs, Medicaid Home and Community-Based Services (HCBS) waivers may provide access to intensive community-based supports, including in-home services, respite care, and case management. However, only a limited number of states offer waivers explicitly inclusive of serious emotional or behavioral disorders, and enrollment caps and waiting lists restrict access even where programs exist (Institute for Families in Society, 2019). As a result, families often rely on piecemeal services across health, education, and child welfare systems, assuming primary responsibility for coordination. The reliance on insurance-based access places a substantial burden on families to navigate eligibility rules, manage appeals, and secure referrals. Children with complex or comorbid mental health conditions frequently fall through gaps between systems, particularly when services are tied to diagnoses or functional thresholds that do not align with fluctuating needs. This fragmentation contributes to delayed care, reliance on emergency services, and significant stress for caregivers (Bitsko et al., 2022).

Canada: Health Care and Mental Health Policy Responses

Canada's universal health care system provides publicly funded access to medically necessary physician and hospital services, including pediatric and adolescent psychiatry Government of Canada, 2025a). In principle, this ensures that children can access diagnostic assessment and physician-led treatment without direct user fees. In practice, access to child and youth mental health services is uneven, with long wait times and substantial variation across provinces and territories (Canadian Institute for Health Information [CIHI], 2023). In Ontario, Canada's most populated province, average wait time is 67 days for counselling and therapy and 92 days for intensive treatment (Children's Mental Health Ontario, 2020).

A central limitation of the Canadian context is the restricted scope of public coverage for non-physician mental health services. Psychotherapy, behavioral interventions, and family-based supports are frequently delivered outside the publicly insured system, requiring private payment or extended health insurance coverage. These gaps create financial barriers for many families, particularly those managing long-term or intensive mental health needs, and contribute to socioeconomic inequities in timely access to care (Signal49 Research, 2023). Direct financial costs alone associated with out-of-pocket expenses are substantial with the average median costs associated with complex care estimated at over $8,639 (Belza et al., 2024).

Provincial and territorial responsibility for health care delivery further contributes to fragmentation. Each jurisdiction establishes its own eligibility criteria, service pathways, and funding priorities for child and youth mental health services. Research consistently documents long waitlists for publicly funded care, limited availability of specialized services for children with complex needs and pronounced geographic disparities between urban and rural areas (Moir et al., 2023).

As a result, families often assume primary responsibility for coordinating services across health, education, and community systems. Qualitative studies describe repeated assessments, multiple entry points, and challenging transitions between services, frequently with limited system-level guidance or continuity (Cleverly, 2025; Stunden et al., 2020).

These coordination burdens are especially pronounced for children with comorbid mental health and neurodevelopmental conditions, whose service needs span multiple sectors and are subject to differing eligibility thresholds. Recent initiatives, such as Integrated Youth Services (IYS) models implemented across Canada, seek to reduce fragmentation by offering coordinated access points for youth mental health services (Canadian Institutes of Health Research, 2023). While early evaluations suggest potential benefits, implementation remains uneven across jurisdictions and does not yet constitute a comprehensive national response.

Overall, Canada's health care system illustrates a pattern of strong universal coverage for physician services combined with fragmented and uneven access to the broader range of supports required by children with mental health disabilities, with significant implications for family burden and service navigation. The German case discussed next illustrates how children's mental health care is structured within a statutory health insurance system, including formal pathways to assessment and treatment.

Germany: Health Care and Mental Health Policy Responses

Germany provides universal health insurance coverage through a statutory health insurance system that covers the majority of the population, including children (Bundesministerium für Gesundheit, 2025a). Mental health services, including child and adolescent psychiatry and psychotherapy, are included within statutory insurance benefits. Coverage is not contingent on income or employment status, reducing financial barriers to access. A defining feature of the German system is the integration of mental health care within broader social insurance frameworks. Child and adolescent mental health services are delivered through a regulated network of providers, with reimbursement rates and service planning overseen through national and regional mechanisms. In contrast to more market-oriented systems, Germany employs needs-based planning to regulate provider distribution, aiming to ensure geographic equity in access. While the German system offers a more structured and comprehensive framework for recognizing and supporting mental health-related care needs, families may still encounter delays in accessing specialized services due to provider shortages and administrative processes. Standardized assessment procedures, while enhancing equity and formal recognition, can also introduce rigidity that may be challenging for families managing fluctuating or episodic mental health conditions.

Germany's statutory health insurance system offers broader formal coverage of mental health services, contributing to comparatively higher baseline uptake.

However, standardized planning mechanisms, workforce shortages, and administrative processes continue to shape when and how care is accessed. While families face fewer direct financial barriers, uptake is still influenced by assessment procedures and provider availability, underscoring that administrative design can shape access even in universal systems. For example, a 2024 study reported that only 34% of children and youth receive a first appointment within four weeks of requesting one and only 54% with a therapeutic need receive actual ongoing care after this first appointment. On average, children and youth waited for 28 weeks to receive therapeutic care (BiPsyMonitor, 2024).

Part 3: Education Systems and Early Childhood Policies

Education systems are central sites for the identification, accommodation, and ongoing support of children with mental health disabilities. Schools often serve as the primary point at which mental health needs are recognized, accommodations are negotiated, and supports are implemented on a day-to-day basis. As such, education policy plays a critical role in shaping how families navigate mental health disability over time, particularly in relation to eligibility determination, enforcement of supports, and coordination across health, education, and community systems.

This section documents how education systems in the United States, Canada, and Germany structure access to educational supports for children with mental health disabilities. The focus is on how eligibility is defined, how accommodations are provided or enforced, and the degree to which families are required to advocate for and monitor supports within educational settings.

United States: Education Policy and Mental Health Disability

In the United States, educational support for children with mental health disabilities is governed by federal civil rights and education statutes, primarily the Individuals with Disabilities Education Act (IDEA) and Section 504 of the Rehabilitation Act. These laws establish enforceable rights to evaluation, accommodation, and services for eligible students nationwide, although implementation varies across states and school districts. Under IDEA, students qualify for special education services if they fall within one of thirteen disability categories and require specially designed instruction. Mental health disabilities are most commonly addressed under the categories of emotional disturbance or other health impairment, depending on how symptoms affect educational performance (National Center for Learning Disabilities, 2024). Eligibility is determined through multidisciplinary evaluation focused on functional impact rather than diagnosis alone. Students found eligible receive an Individualized Education Program (IEP) that specifies goals, accommodations, and related services.

Section 504 provides a parallel civil rights framework for students whose mental health conditions substantially limit one or more major life activities, including learning, but who do not require special education. Section 504 plans may include accommodations such as modified workloads, extended testing time, behavioral supports, or access to school-based mental health services. Unlike IDEA, Section 504 does not guarantee specialized instruction, but it does require schools to provide equal access and prevent discrimination.

Despite these statutory protections, peer-reviewed research documents substantial variability in identification and service provision for students with mental health conditions. Children with internalizing disorders, such as anxiety and depression, are significantly less likely to be identified or to receive school-based supports compared to students with externalizing behaviors, even when functional impairment is comparable (Bradshaw et al., 2008). Families frequently report delays in evaluation, inconsistent implementation of accommodations, and the need for sustained advocacy to secure services, particularly in under-resourced districts (Burke et al., 2017; Du Paul et al., 2020). Early intervention services under IDEA Part C (birth to age three) and preschool services under Part B are intended to support early identification and treatment. However, research indicates that mental health concerns are often under-identified in early childhood settings, and access to evidence-based early childhood mental health interventions remains uneven across states (U.S. Government Accountability Office, 2023). From a policy design perspective, the U.S. education system combines strong formal rights with substantial variation in implementation, shifting monitoring and enforcement responsibilities onto families.

Canada: Education Policy and Mental Health Disability

In Canada, educational supports for students with mental health disabilities are governed through provincial inclusive education frameworks and human rights-based duties to accommodate disability, rather than through a single national education statute (Bennett, 2020). Across provinces and territories, students with mental health disabilities are entitled to accommodation when a disability substantially interferes with learning or participation, although the processes through which needs are identified and supports are provided vary by jurisdiction and school board. Eligibility for educational supports is typically determined through school-based assessment processes that emphasize functional impact rather than diagnosis, allowing flexibility but also introducing discretion at the local level (Bennett, 2020). As a result, access to accommodations often depends on parental advocacy and negotiation with schools, particularly for students with less visible, episodic, or comorbid mental health conditions (Kourgiantakis et al., 2023; Mental Health Commission of Canada, 2023). While this approach aligns with inclusive education principles and avoids rigid categorical labeling, it can also produce uneven implementation and place sustained monitoring and coordination responsibilities on families.

Germany: Education Policy and Mental Health Disability

Germany's education system reflects its federal structure and conservative-corporatist welfare regime, with authority shared between federal and state (Länder) governments. Education policy for children with disabilities is shaped by the Federal Participation Act (Bundesteilhabegesetz) and Germany's obligations under the UN Convention on the Rights of Persons with Disabilities (CRPD), which emphasize participation and inclusion. In practice, Germany maintains a dual system consisting of inclusive education in mainstream schools and specialized schools (Förderschule). Placement decisions are made at the state level based on formal assessments of support needs. Children with mental health disabilities may attend mainstream schools with additional supports or be placed in specialized schools focusing on emotional and social development, depending on severity and available resources (Kultusministerkonferenz, 2018).

BOX 8.1 FÖRDERSCHULEN

In 2016, about 4% of students were enrolled in Förderschulen, only about 0.5% of these students' support needs were identified as emotional or social in nature (Kultusministerkonferenz, 2018). A total of about 40% of students with support needs were enrolled in regular schools and 56% of these students were identified as having social or emotional support needs. When comparing the different support categories across types of schools, students with emotional or social support needs were more likely to be enrolled in regular schools (24%) than in special education schools (12%).

United Nations monitoring bodies have noted ongoing challenges in Germany related to the implementation of inclusive education for children with psychosocial and mental health disabilities, particularly where parallel systems of special schooling persist (United Nations, 2023). Germany provides structured educational supports such as Schulbegleitung (individual school aides) for students requiring assistance with emotional regulation, behavioral support, or daily functioning during the school day. These supports are government funded and are linked to formal assessments of functional limitation (Sozialgesetzbuch [SGB] VIII). Recent scholarly research and government evaluations indicate that while Germany's system offers clearer pathways to formal support than more decentralized systems, families may experience rigidity and administrative burden associated with standardized assessment procedures, particularly for children with fluctuating mental health needs (Powell et al., 2016; United Nations, 2023). Germany's early childhood education system provides a legal entitlement to child care from age one for all children. Unfortunately, most states still provide an insufficient number of spaces to meet the demand. According to the Institute of the German Economy (Institut der deutschen Wirtschaft, 2025) about 14% of children under age three do not have access to needed child care. This number varies from state to state, rising to 18% in Nordrhein Westfalen. The Federal Participation Act also regulates inclusive access to child care, and options include individual support in a regular day care, an inclusive day care or Förderkindergärten (special day care) that provide specialized services for disabled children (Aktion Mensch, 2025). Access to specialized mental health services varies by region and requires navigation of administrative processes (OECD, 2023).

Part 4: Financial Supports, Leave Policies, and Income Security

Financial supports, leave entitlements, and income protection policies play a central role in shaping how families manage the economic dimensions of caring for a child with a mental health disability. Because caregiving associated with children's mental health needs is often long-term, episodic, and unpredictable, policies designed around short-term illness or narrowly defined disability categories may not align well with family circumstances. This section documents how income supports, caregiving leave, and related financial protections are structured in the United States, Canada, and Germany, with attention to eligibility criteria, benefit design, and administrative pathways. Comparative analysis of implications for family burden and equity is addressed in the chapter's concluding synthesis.

United States: Fragmented Income Supports and Limited Financial Protection

In the United States, financial support for families raising children with mental health disabilities is characterized by a fragmented mix of means-tested programs, tax-based benefits, and employer-linked protections. There is no universal caregiving allowance or paid family leave program at the federal level, resulting in significant reliance on household income, employment status, and state-level policy variation.

Income Support and Disability Benefits

Children with severe mental health disabilities may qualify for Supplemental Security Income (SSI), a means-tested cash benefit administered by the Social Security Administration. Eligibility is contingent on strict income and asset limits and on demonstrating marked and severe functional limitations. While SSI can provide a stable source of income for some families, research indicates that many children with significant mental health needs do not receive SSI benefits with great variation across states (Hoagwood et al., 2017). Families may also access Medicaid through SSI eligibility or other pathways, which can reduce medical costs but does not address income loss associated with caregiving demands. Importantly, SSI benefits are modest and rarely sufficient to offset lost earnings or additional caregiving-related expenses. For example, Parish and colleagues found that SSI receipt was significantly associated with improved economic outcomes, but that these improvements were partial and insufficient to eliminate hardship (see, e.g., Parish & Cloud, 2006).

Leave Policies and Employment Protection

The primary federal leave protection available to caregivers is the Family and Medical Leave Act (FMLA), which provides up to 12 weeks of unpaid, job-protected leave for eligible employees. FMLA coverage is limited to workers in firms with at least 50 employees who meet minimum tenure and hours requirements, excluding a substantial proportion of low-wage and part-time workers (U.S. Department of Labor, 2025). Because the leave is unpaid, many families cannot afford to use it, particularly for ongoing or recurrent caregiving needs associated with children's mental health conditions. There is also no federal requirement for employers to provide paid sick leave to parents. As of 2025, 14 states have enacted paid family and medical leave programs that include caregiving for children with serious health conditions, including mental health conditions and 20 states have paid sick leave policies, which include time off for a child's care needs. However, benefit levels, eligibility criteria, and duration vary, resulting in unequal financial protection across states (National Conference of State Legislatures, 2025). For example, the weekly wage replacement rates ranged from $1,000 and $1,600 or between 60 and 100% (New America, 2025).

Canada: Financial Supports and Income Protection

In Canada, financial supports for families raising children with mental health disabilities are provided through a combination of universal child benefits, disability-related supplements, tax-based measures, and employment-linked leave programs (see Tables 8.2 and 8.3). These supports are administered through a mix of federal and provincial programs, resulting in multiple entry points and varied eligibility requirements (Government of Canada, 2024). While this policy architecture offers broad coverage in principle, access to specific benefits often depends on administrative classification, employment attachment, and the ability to navigate complex application processes (Finlay et al., 2023). A recent report on the state of disability policy for children in Canada finds 78% of parents reported difficulty applying for disability programs with identified barriers attributed to administrative complexity, unclear eligibility criteria, and lack of system guidance (Finlay et al., 2023).

Key federal income support for families is the Disability Tax Credit which functions as a gateway to multiple federal benefits (Finlay et al., 2023). Eligibility for the DTC is determined through medical certification of prolonged and marked functional impairment (Government of Canada, 2025b). Policy analyses and linked administrative data indicate that families of children with mental health and neurodevelopmental disabilities face particular challenges qualifying for the DTC due to the episodic, fluctuating, or less visible nature of these conditions, contributing to lower uptake relative to potential eligibility (Leanage et al., 2025). As a result, access to disability-related income supports may be uneven even among families experiencing substantial caregiving demands (Leanage et al., 2025).

Employment-linked caregiving supports are primarily delivered through the federal Employment Insurance (EI) system, which provides time-limited caregiving benefits under specific conditions. These benefits are designed primarily for acute or time-bound care episodes and are contingent on recent labor force attachment, excluding some caregivers whose employment has already been disrupted by caregiving responsibilities (ESDC, 2023). Research on caregiving and employment in Canada suggests that parents managing long-term mental health–related caregiving are less likely to meet eligibility requirements and less likely to use EI caregiving benefits when care needs are ongoing or episodic rather than crisis-based (Cai et al., 2025; Lero et al., 2017).

Taken together, Canada's income support and leave policies illustrate a system that combines broad-based family benefits with disability-specific and employment-contingent programs. The interaction of these programs shapes the extent to which families can offset income loss, manage care-related expenses, and remain attached to the labor market over time (Finlay et al., 2023; Leanage et al., 2025).

Germany: Formal Recognition of Caregiving and Structured Income Protection

Germany offers the most comprehensive and structured system of financial support for caregiving among the three countries examined. Financial protections are embedded within social insurance frameworks that explicitly recognize caregiving as a social responsibility.

Long-term Care Insurance and Cash Benefits

Germany's long-term care insurance (Pflegeversicherung) provides cash benefits (Pflegegeld) and in-kind services to individuals with recognized care needs, which since 2017 also includes children with mental health disabilities when impairments substantially limit daily functioning. It can be more challenging to communicate the care needs for a mental health disability compared to more visible physical care needs, which can make it more difficult to receive a care level (Agentur für Haushaltshilfe, n.d.). Care levels (Pflegegrade) are determined through standardized assessments that consider psychological and cognitive impairments alongside physical needs (Bundesministerium für Gesundheit, 2017). Families caring for eligible children may receive monthly cash benefits that partially compensate for caregiving labor or pay for support services. Unlike means-tested programs, eligibility is not contingent on income, reducing economic exclusion.

BOX 8.2 CARE INSURANCE

There are 5 different care levels with higher care levels representing greater impairment and greater need for support. The benefit type and amount received by families varies depending on the Pflegegrad (Bundesministerium für Gesundheit, 2017). At care level one, families can only receive 125 euros Entlastunsbeitrag, a reimbursement for specific services used to manage care such as short-term in-patient care, respite care, or support with household chores. They can also receive 4,000 euros for necessary modifications to their home. If an individual receives care level 2–5 and is cared for in their own home, they are eligible for a cash benefit and additional funding to pay for equipment or in-home nursing services. Depending on the level of care, the cash benefit ranges from 316 to 901 euros, and the funding for services and equipment ranges from 689 to 1,995 euros. In 2024, care insurance paid 63 billion Euros in benefits to around 6 million people, mainly to finance in-home or outpatient care (Bundesministerium für Gesundheit, 2025f).

Caregiving Leave and Employment Protection

Germany provides multiple statutory leave options for caregivers, including short-term emergency leave and longer-term unpaid or partially compensated leave arrangements. Caregiving leave laws allow parents to reduce working hours or take leave while maintaining job protection, and social insurance contributions may continue during caregiving periods (Bundesministerium für Gesundheit, 2025b). These provisions reduce the risk of permanent labor market exit and mitigate long-term income loss associated with caregiving. Despite these protections, a gender care gap remains with 80% of mothers caring for a disabled child being the main care provider and being more likely to reduce employment hours (50.6%) or stop work altogether (26.2%; Kofahl & Lüdecke, 2014).

BOX 8.3 LEAVE POLICIES

There are a variety of different leave programs available for families in Germany. All birthing mothers are entitled to leave four weeks before and eight weeks after delivery. Paid parental leave is available for either 14 or 32 months with varying payments for birth and adoptive parents (Bundesministerium für Bildung, Familie, Senioren, Frauen und Jugend, 2025) and unpaid leave for up to three years. Based on the Pflegezeitgesetz family members can take a full or partial leave from work for up to six months to take care of a family member including children either in the home or in a facility, for example in case of a longer hospital stay. The Familienpflegezeitgesetz allows for up to 24 months of unpaid partial leave and it is limited to employers with at least 25 employees. Employees also have to work for at least 15 hours per week to be eligible for this partial leave.

Part 5: Anti-Discrimination Policies

Anti-discrimination legislation shapes whether and how parents of children with mental health disabilities and their parents are protected from differential treatment in employment and other institutional settings. Such protections determine the extent to which caregiving responsibilities are recognized as legitimate grounds for accommodation and whether families can assert rights without fear of retaliation or job loss. This section documents the structure of anti-discrimination frameworks relevant to caregiving and disability in the United States, Canada, and Germany, with attention to the scope of protected grounds, mechanisms for enforcement, and the administrative processes families must navigate to access protections. The implications of these frameworks for family security, caregiving burden, and social work practice are addressed in the chapter's concluding synthesis.

United States: Protections in the Workplace

There are a variety of different policies that protect employees from discrimination in the workplace. In this section we would like to mention specific policies that apply most closely to exceptional care and workplace discrimination, since family members might experience discrimination in the workplace due to their family care responsibilities or family responsibility discrimination (FRD) (Work Life Law, 2025). There is no federal policy that protects employees from discrimination based on their care responsibilities, but over 200 cities have protections specific to family responsibilities (Work Life Law, 2025). Unfortunately, only a handful of states have explicit protections against family responsibility discrimination. In the case of caring for a child with a mental health disability, families are also protected against workplace discrimination through provisions of the Americans with Disabilities Act (ADA, 1990), since the ADA also prohibits discrimination against anyone associated with a disabled person, which would include parents of a child with a mental health disability (Work Life Law, 2025). Employed parents are not just protected against discrimination, but they have a right to reasonable accommodations just like employees with disabilities. For example, if it does not create undue hardship for the employer, employees have to be allowed to work remotely to be able to care for their disabled child.

Canada: Anti-Discrimination Protections Related to Caregiving and Disability

In Canada, protections against discrimination related to disability and caregiving are grounded in a combination of federal and provincial human rights legislation. At the federal level, the Canadian Human Rights Act prohibits discrimination on the basis of disability and family status in federally regulated employment and services (Canadian Human Rights Act, R.S.C. 1985, c. H-6). All provinces and territories similarly prohibit disability-based discrimination under their respective human rights codes, including association-based discrimination, which extends protection to individuals who experience adverse treatment because of their relationship to a person with a disability.

Several provincial statutes explicitly recognize family status as a protected ground, including the Ontario Human Rights Code (1990), the British Columbia Human Rights Code (Human Rights Code, 1996), and the Alberta Human Rights Act (Alberta Human Rights Act, RSA 2000, c A-25.5). Canadian courts have increasingly recognized that workplace rules that significantly interfere with caregiving responsibilities may constitute discrimination based on family status (Health Sciences Association of British Columbia v. Campbell River and North Island Transition Society, 2004; *Canada (Attorney General) v. Johnstone*, 2014). However, the scope of family status protections and the threshold for establishing a duty to accommodate vary across jurisdictions and have been shaped largely through tribunal and court decisions rather than through uniform statutory definitions (Vipond & Oliphant, 2020).

In practice, enforcement of these protections relies on individual, complaint-based processes. Parents seeking accommodation or redress must initiate claims through human rights commissions or tribunals, demonstrate prima facie discrimination, and engage in adjudicative procedures that can be lengthy and adversarial. Research and policy analyses indicate that these procedural requirements can limit access to protection for families already experiencing significant caregiving and employment strain, particularly when discrimination is subtle, episodic, or tied to mental health–related stigma rather than overt exclusion (Vipond & Oliphant, 2020). As a result, while Canada's human rights framework provides formal legal protection against discrimination related to disability and caregiving, the extent to which these protections translate into practical workplace security depends heavily on families' capacity to navigate legal and administrative systems.

Germany: Protections in the Workplace

Since December 2022 with changes to the employment anti-discrimination legislation in Germany, employees who suspect discrimination based on family care responsibilities can reach out to the federal anti-discrimination office (Antidiskriminierungsstelle des Bundes, 2025). A 2025 decision of the European Court also confirmed that working parents of children with disabilities enjoy the same anti-discrimination protections as disabled employees. They accordingly also have a right to workplace accommodations to integrate both work and care responsibilities (Hyseni, 2025). Employed parents caring for a child with a mental health disability might therefore be protected from discrimination both based on protections against discrimination based on care responsibilities and based on the disability status.

The preceding sections demonstrate that families raising children with mental health disabilities encounter distinct but interrelated policy environments across health care, education, financial supports, and anti-discrimination frameworks. Each domain structures access, eligibility, and responsibility in different ways, often requiring families to navigate multiple systems simultaneously as children's needs evolve over time. While these policy areas are typically governed separately, families experience them as interconnected, with gaps or constraints in one domain frequently amplifying uncertainty and burden in others. The following section brings these policy domains into conversation, synthesizing cross-national evidence to examine how institutional design across sectors shapes caregiving trajectories, allocates risk between families and the state, and creates implications for social work practice and policy development.

Part 6: Cross-Domain Synthesis and Policy Implications: A Disability Rights Perspective

Welfare regime theory is used in this chapter to explain cross-national differences in policy design and how these differences structure parents' ability to navigate formal services and supports for children with mental health disabilities (Bambra, 2007; Esping-Andersen, 1990). To interpret the implications of these policy designs for families' capacity to realize rights in practice, the analysis draws on disability rights principles. Examining health care, education, financial supports, and anti-discrimination frameworks in the United States, Canada, and Germany highlights that children's mental health disability is not only a clinical or educational concern, but a core social welfare and disability rights issue shaped by institutional arrangements. Consistent with the United Nations Convention on the Rights of Persons with Disabilities (CRPD), disability rights are realized not through formal recognition alone, but through effective access, meaningful participation, and reasonable accommodation across social systems (United Nations, 2006). From this perspective, the central issue is not whether children's mental health needs are acknowledged in principle, but whether policy arrangements reduce uncertainty for families and enable rights to be exercised without requiring sustained navigation, advocacy, or crisis-driven intervention.

Although all three countries are high-income democracies with high levels of human development, they differ markedly in how responsibility for children's mental health care and associated caregiving labor is allocated among families, the state, and the market. Grounded in welfare regime theory (Bambra, 2007; Esping-Andersen, 1990), the analysis demonstrates that cross-national differences in family experiences are best understood not as failures of individual systems, but as predictable consequences of regime-specific policy logics that either facilitate or constrain the realization of disability rights in everyday practice. Where policy frameworks rely on fragmented services, conditional eligibility, or reactive enforcement, families are left to navigate uncertainty across systems, effectively bearing responsibility for translating formal rights into lived support.

Health Care: Effective Access and Continuity of Support

Access to timely and appropriate health care is foundational to participation in education, family life, and community (UNCRDP, 2026). Across all three countries, children's mental health needs are formally recognized within health care systems, yet access and continuity are shaped by how services are financed, organized, and integrated. In the United States, reliance on insurance-based access exposes families to financial risk and variable service availability, limiting the extent to which access functions as a right rather than a contingent benefit (Beronio et al., 2013; Foster et al., 2026). Canada's universal physician coverage supports diagnostic access but leaves many therapeutic and community-based services outside public insurance, separating recognition of need from the provision of ongoing support (Kourgiantakis et al., 2023; Waddell et al., 2018). Germany's statutory insurance model offers stronger formal recognition, yet standardized assessments and capacity constraints can restrict continuity for children with episodic or fluctuating conditions (Robert Koch Institute, 2022).

Across contexts, these arrangements illustrate a common gap between formal entitlement and effective access. Where systems lack sufficient capacity or integrated care pathways, families become de facto coordinators of care, navigating uncertainty despite nominal coverage. From a disability rights standpoint, such arrangements fall short of ensuring access on an equal basis with others, as envisioned under the CRPD.

Education: Participation, Accommodation, and Enforcement

Education systems are central to the realization of children's rights to participation and inclusion under the CRPD. In the United States, enforceable rights under IDEA and Section 504 establish a strong legal framework, but uneven implementation and under-identification of internalizing mental health conditions limit consistent access to accommodations (Bradshaw et al., 2008; DuPaul et al., 2019). Canada's inclusive education orientation and functional assessment processes align with rights-based principles, yet reliance on provincial discretion and school-level decision-making often conditions access on parental advocacy (Bennett et al., 2018; People for Education, 2024). Germany provides more structured supports, including individualized assistance, but continues to balance inclusive education with parallel systems, reflecting ongoing tensions between participation and differentiation (Powell et al., 2016; Kultusministerkonferenz, 2018).

From a disability rights perspective, education systems that depend on sustained parental advocacy to secure accommodations effectively privatize enforcement of rights. When access to reasonable accommodation hinges on family capacity rather than institutional obligation, uncertainty becomes a defining feature of families' experiences, undermining children's right to inclusive and predictable educational participation.

Financial Supports: Shared Responsibility and Recognition of Caregiving

The CRPD emphasizes the role of social protection in enabling families to support children with disabilities without disproportionate hardship. Financial and income support policies therefore provide a critical lens on how caregiving is recognized and whether responsibility is shared. In the United States, reliance on means-tested benefits and employer-linked leave exposes families to economic insecurity, constraining their ability to sustain care over time (Parish & Cloud, 2006). Canada's broader family benefits offer partial protection, but disability-related supports and caregiving leave remain contingent on administrative classification and employment attachment, limiting their effectiveness for families managing long-term mental health needs (Cai et al., 2025). Germany's social insurance model more explicitly recognizes caregiving through cash benefits and leave protections, reducing household-level financial risk even when care demands persist (Bundesministerium für Gesundheit, 2017). Despite these protections, the long-term financial impact on individuals when dropping out of the workforce remains in Germany. Care insurance benefits often do not make up for all lost wages, and contributions to retirement will be reduced as well. Overall, viewed through a disability rights lens, policies that formally recognize caregiving as a shared social responsibility reduce uncertainty and enable families to exercise rights without sacrificing economic security. Where recognition is partial or conditional, families absorb the costs of disability-related care through reduced employment, income loss, and long-term precarity.

Anti-Discrimination Legislation: Protection, Accessibility, and Realization of Rights

Anti-discrimination frameworks are essential for protecting parents from adverse treatment related to disability and caregiving responsibilities. Across all three countries, disability is recognized as a protected ground, and some form of association-based protection exists. However, consistent with CRPD principles, the realization of these protections depends on accessibility and enforceability. Complaint-based systems that rely on individual families to initiate legal action place substantial burdens on caregivers already navigating complex systems. While such frameworks signal societal commitment to equality and can deter overt discrimination, their capacity to secure reasonable accommodation is limited when enforcement is reactive, procedurally demanding, and vulnerable to shifts in political priorities or administrative enforcement.

Part 7: Implications for Social Work and Social Welfare Policy

Across domains, the comparative analysis reveals a consistent pattern: policies that recognize children's mental health disability in principle frequently rely on families to navigate uncertainty in practice. Health care systems that fragment access, education systems that condition accommodation on advocacy, financial supports that incompletely recognize caregiving, and anti-discrimination frameworks that depend on individual enforcement collectively shape caregiving as an ongoing process of navigating the unknown.

For social work practice, these findings highlight the profession's central role in translating disability rights into lived access. Social workers are often positioned at the intersections of health, education, and social protection systems, where they support families in navigating eligibility, securing accommodations, and responding to institutional uncertainty. At the policy level, the analysis points to the need for social welfare reforms that align health, education, income, and employment policies with CRPD principles, shifting responsibility from families to institutions and reducing reliance on parental capacity to realize rights. Together, these implications underscore the importance of disability rights–oriented policy design in reducing uncertainty and advancing equitable support for children with mental health disabilities and their families.

Part 8: Summary and Key Points

This chapter examined how national social policy frameworks shape the experiences of families raising children with mental health disabilities across the United States, Canada, and Germany. Using a comparative policy lens grounded in welfare regime theory, the chapter documented how health care systems, education policies, financial supports, and anti-discrimination frameworks structure access to services, allocate responsibility for care, and distribute risk between families and institutions. Across all domains, the analysis demonstrated that children's mental health disability is not solely a clinical or educational concern, but a core social welfare issue shaped by institutional design.

Although all three countries formally recognize children's mental health needs, the chapter showed that recognition alone does not ensure usable access or continuity of support. Differences in policy architecture produce distinct patterns of uncertainty for families, particularly where services are fragmented, eligibility is conditional, or enforcement relies on individual advocacy. Health care systems vary in how they finance and organize mental health services, education systems differ in the enforceability of accommodations and the degree of parental advocacy required, financial supports unevenly recognize caregiving labor, and anti-discrimination protections often depend on complaint-based enforcement. Taken together, these arrangements shape caregiving as an ongoing process of navigating multiple systems rather than a predictable pathway of support.

Viewed through a disability rights perspective informed by the UN Convention on the Rights of Persons with Disabilities, the chapter highlighted a recurring gap between formal policy recognition and the realization of rights in practice. Across countries, families are frequently required to translate rights into access through sustained navigation, coordination, and advocacy, particularly when children's mental health needs are episodic or fluctuate over time. The chapter underscored that these dynamics are not the result of individual system failures, but reflect broader welfare regime logics that condition how responsibility for care is shared between families, the state, and the market.

Part 9: Application for Social Work Education

The following activities can strengthen students' skills in different areas of social work practice.

Activity 1: Comparative policy discussion

Using the resources provided below, students can conduct further research on any of the policy areas discussed above and discuss the following questions:

- What are the differences and similarities between countries?
- How does this policy align with a human rights and social justice framework?
- What are the shortcomings?

Activity 2: Policy analysis

Competency 2: Advance Human Rights and Social, Racial, Economic, and Environmental Justice
Competency 5: Engage in Policy Practice

Based on the information provided in this chapter, students conduct a policy analysis of the health care coverage, educational policies, or anti-discrimination policies, answering the following questions:

- What benefit/service is provided by the program?
- Who is eligible for the benefit?
- How is the program financed?
- Who implements the program?
- Does it reach the intended population, especially when considering the needs of children with mental health disabilities?
- Is everyone covered adequately, especially when considering mental health needs?
- How do the costs compare to the benefits?
- Are there unintended consequences?
- Is it aligned with social justice?

Activity 3: Application to family case

Competency 8: Intervene with Individuals, Families, Groups, Organizations, and Communities

Based on the experiences of family Lopez introduced in chapter 4, discuss how their experience and your intervention might change if they lived in Canada or Germany.

Julia (mother, 42), Robert (father, 47), Maria (daughter, 12), and Ben (son, 10). Hunter just moved to a new state, because Robert was offered a better-paying position at a non-profit agency. Julia is currently looking for a new position as an accountant. Money is tighter right now, since Julia is not working. Maria and Ben are both enrolled in public schools, Maria in a large middle school and Ben in a small elementary school. Maria has recently been diagnosed with depression and an eating disorder, which upended the family's routines. Maria participates in an out-patient half-day treatment program. Julia is driving Maria to the clinic at 8 am in the morning and picks her up at 1pm. Robert is helping Ben in the mornings and makes sure he gets on the school bus before heading to work. Maria is not going to school right now and has to be supervised. Maria and Julia spend the afternoon together until they pick up Ben from school. Robert often comes home late from work, since he is still learning his new job. Luckily, Robert's job comes with good health insurance and the out-of-pocket payments for Maria's current treatment is manageable. The family doesn't have friends yet, since they just moved to the new town. Julia and Robert left behind their parents and siblings. While they don't have any family members in the area, they all feel very connected to each other. Ben has been acting out at home and at school. His school has called his parents for a meeting, since Ben hit another schoolmate in a fight over the monkey bars. You are a social worker in Maria's clinic and you work with the family members of the children receiving treatment.

- What are the anti-discrimination policies applicable in Canada or Germany that would protect Robert?
- If Maria required a substantial amount of care, how could care insurance in Germany support this family?
- How would the different health insurance schemes affect Maria's access to treatment?

Resource List

Core Frameworks and Disability Rights

(Foundational texts supporting the chapter's conceptual approach)

Esping-Andersen, G. (1990). *The three worlds of welfare capitalism.* Princeton University Press.
Bambra, C. (2007). Going beyond the three worlds of welfare capitalism. *Journal of Epidemiology & Community Health*, 61(12), 1098–1102.
Shakespeare, T. (2014). *Disability rights and wrongs revisited.* Routledge.
United Nations. (2006). *Convention on the Rights of Persons with Disabilities (CRPD).*

Comparative policy and data sources

(Useful for cross-national policy analysis and student assignments)

OECD. (2021). *A new benchmark for mental health systems.* OECD Publishing.
OECD Family Database. https://www.oecd.org/els/family/database.htm
UNDP Human Development Reports. https://hdr.undp.org

Country-specific policy and system resources

(Authoritative sources referenced throughout the chapter)

United States:

National Survey of Children's Health (NSCH). https://mchb.hrsa.gov/data

Canada:

Canadian Institute for Health Information (CIHI). https://www.cihi.ca
Canadian Centre for Caregiving Excellence (CCCE). https://canadiancaregiving.org

Germany:

Robert Koch Institute (RKI). https://www.rki.de

Practice-oriented resources

(Supporting social work practice, advocacy, and teaching)

International Disability Alliance. https://www.internationaldisabilityalliance.org
Center for WorkLife Law. https://worklifelaw.org

References

Agentur für Haushaltspflege (n.d.). Psychische Erkrankungen: Tipps zum Pflegegrad beantragen https://www.agentur-fuer-haushaltshilfe.de/psychische-erkrankungen-tipps-zum-pflegegrad-beantragen/

Aktion Mensch (2025). Kita für Kinder über 3 Jahre (Ü3). https://www.familienratgeber.de/lebensbereiche/kita-schule/ue3-kita

Alberta Human Rights Act, R.S.A. (2000). c. A-25.5 (Alta.). https://www.canlii.org/en/ab/laws/stat/rsa-2000-c-a-25.5/latest/rsa-2000-c-a-25.5.html?loginActive=true

Americans with Disabilities Act Amendments Act of 2008, 42 U.S.C. § 12102. https://www.law.cornell.edu/uscode/text/42/12102

Antidiskriminierungsstelle des Bundes (2025). Diskriminierung von Eltern und pflegenden Angehörigen im Beruf. https://www.antidiskriminierungsstelle.de/DE/ueber-diskriminierung/lebensbereiche/arbeitsleben/fuersorgende-erwerbstaetige/fuersorgende-erwerbstaetige.html

Bambra, C. (2007). Going beyond the three worlds of welfare capitalism: Regime theory and public health research. *Journal of Epidemiology & Community Health*, *61*(12), 1098–1102. https://doi.org/10.1136/jech.2007.064295

Belza, C., Cohen, E., Orkin, J., Fayed, N., Major, N., Quartarone, S., & Moretti, M. (2024). Out-of-pocket expenses reported by families of children with medical complexity. *Paediatrics & Child Health*, *29*(4), 216–223. https://doi.org/10.1093/pch/pxad040

Bennett, P. W. (2020). *The state of the system: A reality check on Canada's schools*. McGill-Queen's Press – MQUP.

Beronio, K., Po, R., Skopec, L., & Glied, S. (2013). Affordable care act expands mental health and substance use disorder benefits. *Health Affairs*, *32*(6), 1044–1052. https://doi.org/10.1377/hlthaff.2013.0120

BiPsyMonitor (2024). Psychosoziale Versorgungsstrukturen für Kinder und Jugendliche, schulische Belastungsfaktoren und Versorgungsbarrieren: Einblick in erste Ergebnisse aus den Erhebungswellen 2024. https://bipsy.de/wp-content/uploads/Fact-Sheet_Versorgungsmonitor_neues-Design.pdf

Bitsko, R. H., Claussen, A. H., Lichstein, J., et al. (2022). Mental health surveillance among children—United States, 2013–2019. *Morbidity and Mortality Weekly Report Supplements*, *71*(2), 1–42. https://doi.org/10.15585/mmwr.su7102a1

Bradshaw, C. P., Buckley, J. A., & Ialongo, N. S. (2008). School-based service utilization among urban children with early onset educational and mental health problems: The squeaky wheel phenomenon. *School Psychology Quarterly*, *23*(2), 169–186. https://doi.org/10.1037/1045-3830.23.2.169

Bundesministerium für Gesundheit (2017). Die Pflegestärkungsgesetze. Alle Leistungen zum Nachschlagen. https://www.bundesgesundheitsministerium.de/fileadmin/Dateien/5_Publikationen/Pflege/Broschueren/PSG_Alle_Leistungen.pdf

Bundesministerium für Gesundheit (2025a). Gesetzliche Krankenversicherung. https://www.bundesgesundheitsministerium.de/gkv.html

Bundesministerium für Gesundheit (2025b). Wie wird die Vereinbarkeit von Pflege und Beruf gefördert. https://www.bundesgesundheitsministerium.de/themen/pflege/online-ratgeber-pflege/leistungen-der-pflegeversicherung/leistungen-im-ueberblick/wie-wird-die-vereinbarkeit-von-pflege-und-beruf-gefoerdert.html

Burke, M. M., Meadan-Kaplansky, H., Patton, K. A., Pearson, J. N., Cummings, K. P., & Lee, C. eun. (2018). Advocacy for children with social-communication needs: Perspectives from parents and school professionals. *The Journal of Special Education*, *51*(4), 191–200. https://doi.org/10.1177/0022466917716898

Cai, M., Lero, D., & Fuller, S. (2025). *Care/work policies for managing routine and unpredictable caregiving* (Policy brief). The Vanier Institute of the Family. https://doi.org/10.61959/ESNT2797E

Canada (Attorney General) v. Johnstone (2014). FCA 110 (CanLII). https://www.canlii.org/en/ca/fca/doc/2014/2014fca110/2014fca110.html

Canadian Human Rights Act, R.S.C. (1985), c. H-6 (Can.). https://laws-lois.justice.gc.ca/eng/acts/h-6/

Canadian Human Rights Commission. (2026). *Duty to accommodate*. https://www.chrc-ccdp.gc.ca/individuals/human-rights/duty-accommodate

Canadian Institute for Health Information. (2025). Child and youth mental health in Canada. https://www.cihi.ca/en/child-and-youth-mental-health

Canadian Institutes of Health Research. (2023, November 28). *IYS-Net: About*. Government of Canada. https://cihr-irsc.gc.ca/e/52913.html

Children's Mental Health Ontario. (2020). *Kids can't wait: 2020 report on wait times for child and youth mental health services in Ontario*. https://cmho.org/wp-content/uploads/CMHO-Report-WaitTimes-2020.pdf

Cleverley, K., Salman, S., Ewing, L., Davies, J., Ang, H., Daley, M., Brennenstuhl, S., Nasir, S., Lemke, K., Charach, A., Monga, S., & Korczak, D. (2026). Evaluation of the mental health transition navigation model in child and adolescent mental health settings: Findings from a pre-post, mixed-methods study. *European Child & Adolescent Psychiatry*, *35*(2), 599–610. https://doi.org/10.1007/s00787-025-02872-w

DuPaul, G. J., Chronis-Tuscano, A., Danielson, M. L., & Visser, S. N. (2019). Predictors of receipt of school services in a national sample of youth with ADHD. *Journal of Attention Disorders*, *23*(11), 1303–1319. https://doi.org/10.1177/1087054718816169

Esping-Andersen, G. (1990). *The three worlds of welfare capitalism*. Princeton University Press.

Finlay, B., Ragot, S., Lach, L. M., & Zwicker, J. D. (2023). *Disability policy in Canada: Federal report*. Kids Brain Health Network. https://kidsbrainhealth.ca/wp-content/uploads/2023/11/Disability-Policy-in-Canada-Federal-Report-Final_Nov27.pdf

Foster, A. A., Cushing, A. M., Hoffmann, J. A., Nash, K. A., Lee, C. M., & Michelson, K. A. (2026). Expenditures for pediatric behavioral health care over time and estimated family financial burden. *JAMA Pediatrics*, *180*(2), 194–201. https://doi.org/10.1001/jamapediatrics.2025.5181

Government of Canada. (2022). Evaluation of the Employment Insurance Parents of Critically Ill Children benefit. https://www.canada.ca/en/employment-social-development/corporate/reports/evaluations/parents-critically-ill-children-benefit.html

Government of Canada. (2024). Employment insurance caregiving benefits. https://www.canada.ca/en/services/benefits/ei/caregiving/eligibility.html

Government of Canada. (2025a). About Canada's health care system. Government of Canada. https://www.canada.ca/en/health-canada/services/canada-health-care-system.html

Government of Canada (2025b). Disability tax credit. https://www.canada.ca/en/revenue-agency/services/tax/individuals/segments/tax-credits-deductions-persons-disabilities/disability-tax-credit/eligible-dtc.html

Health Sciences Association of British Columbia v. Campbell River and North Island Transition Society, 2004 BCCA 260 (CanLII). https://www.canlii.org/en/bc/bcca/doc/2004/2004bcca260/2004bcca260.html

Hoagwood, K. E., Zima, B. T., Buka, S. L., Houtrow, A., & Kelleher, K. J. (2017). State-to-state variation in SSI enrollment for children with mental disabilities: An administrative and ethical challenge. *Psychiatric Services, 68*(2), 195–198. https://doi.org/10.1176/appi.ps.201600118

Human Resources and Skills Development Canada. (2013). *Federal disability reference guide* (ISSD-091-06-13E). Government of Canada. https://www.canada.ca/content/dam/esdc-edsc/migration/documents/eng/disability/arc/reference_guide.pdf

Hyseni, E. (2025). Pflege eines Kindes mit Behinderung muss möglich sein. Tagesschau. https://www.tagesschau.de/wirtschaft/arbeitsmarkt/eugh-urteil-diskriminierung-eltern-behinderung-kind-100.html

Individuals with Disabilities Education Act, 20 U.S.C. § 1401. https://www.congress.gov/111/plaws/publ256/PLAW-111publ256.pdf

Institut der deutschen Wirtschaft (2025). Kinderbetreuung: 300.000 Kitaplätze für unter Dreijährige fehlen https://www.iwkoeln.de/presse/pressemitteilungen/wido-geis-thoene-300000-kitplaetze-fuer-unter-dreijaehrige-fehlen.html

Kofahl, C. & Lüdecke, D. (2014). Familie im Fokus – Die Lebens- und Versorgungssituation von Familien mit chronisch kranken und behinderten Kindern in Deutschland. Ergebnisse der Kindernetzwerk-Studie. Abteilung Prävention des AOK-Bundesverbandes. https://www.bvktp.de/media/aok-bv_33selbsthilfestudie_web.pdf

Kourgiantakis, T., Markoulakis, R., Lee, E., Hussain, A., Lau, C., & Ashcroft, R. (2023). Access to mental health and addiction services for youth and families in Ontario. *International Journal of Mental Health Systems, 17*, Article 4. https://doi.org/10.1186/s13033-023-00572-z

Leanage, A., Jeon, S.-H., & Arim, R. (2025). Uptake of the disability tax credit and CPP/QPP disability benefits. *Statistics Canada Economic and Social Reports*. https://doi.org/10.25318/36280001202500200001-eng

Lero, D. S., Spinks, N., Fast, J., Hilbrecht, M., & Tremblay, D. (2017). *The availability, accessibility and effectiveness of workplace supports for Canadian caregivers*. University of Guelph, Centre for Families, Work & Well-Being.

Leung, B. M. Y., Wandler, C., Pringsheim, T., & Santana, M. J. (2022). Working with parents of children with complex mental health issues. *Journal of Child Health Care, 26*(4), 548–567. https://doi.org/10.1177/13674935211028694

Lynch, F., & Dickerson, J. (2012). PS2-21: Validity and reliability of the family economic impact interview: A new instrument to measure costs related to child mental health conditions. *Clinical Medical Research, 10*(3), 1–81.

Mental Health Commission of Canada. (2023, January). *Brave new world: Integrated service hubs are transforming youth mental health care in Canada.* https://mentalhealthcommission.ca/catalyst/brave-new-world/

Moir, M., Barua, B., & with Wannamaker, H. (2023). *Waiting your turn: Wait times for health care in Canada, 2023 report*. Fraser Institute. https://www.fraserinstitute.org/studies/waiting-your-turn-wait-times-for-health-care-in-canada-2023

National Center for Health Workforce Analysis. (2024). State of the behavioral health workforce. Retrieved from: https://bhw.hrsa.gov/sites/default/files/bureau-health-workforce/state-of-the-behavioral-health-workforce-report-2024.pdf

National Center for Learning Disabilities. (2024). IEPs vs. 504 plans. https://ncld.org/ieps-vs-504-plans/

National Conference of State Legislatures. (2025). Paid leave: State Family and Medical Leave Laws https://www.ncsl.org/labor-and-employment/state-family-and-medical-leave-laws

Ontario Human Rights Commission. (2014). *Policy on preventing discrimination based on mental health disabilities and addictions*. https://www3.ohrc.on.ca/en/policy-preventing-discrimination-based-mental-health-disabilities-and-addictions

Organization for Economic Co-operation and Development. (2021). *A new benchmark for mental health systems: Tackling the social and economic costs of mental ill-health.* OECD Publishing. https://doi.org/10.1787/4ed890f6-en

Organization for Economic Co-operation and Development. (2024). *OECD economic outlook.* https://www.oecd.org/economic-outlook/

Parish, S. L., & Cloud, J. M. (2006). Financial well-being of young children with disabilities and their families. *Social Work, 51*(3), 223–232. https://doi.org/10.1093/sw/51.3.223

Peters, C. P. (2006). EPSDT: Medicaid's critical but controversial benefits program for children. Washington (DC): National Health Policy Forum https://www.ncbi.nlm.nih.gov/books/NBK560010/

Polanczyk, G. V., Salum, G. A., Sugaya, L. S., Caye, A., & Rohde, L. A. (2022). Annual research review: A meta-analysis of the worldwide prevalence of mental disorders in children and adolescents. *Journal of Child Psychology and Psychiatry, 63*(4), 431–440. https://doi.org/10.1111/jcpp.13554

Powell, J. J. W., Edelstein, B., & Blanck, J. M. (2016). Awareness raising, legitimation or backlash? Effects of the UN Convention on the Rights of Persons with Disabilities on education systems in Germany. *Globalisation, Societies and Education, 14*(2), 227–250. http://dx.doi.org/10.1080/14767724.2014.982076

Robert Koch Institute. (2022). Psychische Gesundheit in Deutschland. https://www.rki.de/DE/Themen/Nichtuebertragbare-Krankheiten/Psychische-Gesundheit/Psychische-Gesundheit-und-Stoerungen/EBH_Bericht_Psyschiche_Gesundheit-Teil2.pdf?__blob=publicationFile&v=1

Signal49 Research. (2023). *The health and economic imperative for investing in children's healthcare*. https://www.signal49.ca/wp-content/uploads/2022/10/the-health-imperitive_childrens-healthcare_2023.pdf

Sozialgesetzbuch (SGB) IX – Rehabilitation und Teilhabe von Menschen mit Behinderungen, § 2 (Ger.). https://www.gesetze-im-internet.de/sgb_9/

Sozialgesetzbuch (SGB) VIII - § 35a SGB VIII Eingliederungshilfe für Kinder und Jugendliche mit seelischer Behinderung oder drohender seelischer Behinderung. https://www.sozialgesetzbuch-sgb.de/sgbviii/35a.html

Stunden, C., Zasada, J., VanHeerwaarden, N., Hollenberg, E., Abi-Jaoudé, A., Chaim, G., Cleverley, K., Henderson, J., Johnson, A., Levinson, A., Lo, B., Robb, J., Shi, J., Voineskos, A., & Wiljer, D. (2020). Help-seeking behaviors of transition-aged youth for mental health concerns: Qualitative study. *Journal of Medical Internet Research, 22*(10), e18514. https://doi.org/10.2196/18514

U.S. Department of Labor. (2025). Family and Medical Leave Act. https://www.dol.gov/agencies/whd/fmla

U.S. Government Accountability Office (2023). Special education: Additional data could help early intervention programs reach more eligible infants and toddlers. Retrieved from: https://www.gao.gov/assets/gao-24-106019.pdf

United Nations. (2006). *Convention on the rights of persons with disabilities*. https://www.un.org/development/desa/disabilities/convention-on-the-rights-of-persons-with-disabilities.html

United Nations. (2023). *Concluding observations on the combined second and third periodic reports of Germany*. https://digitallibrary.un.org/record/4023219?v=pdf

United Nations Development Program. (2023). *Human development report 2023/2024*. https://hdr.undp.org

Vipond, M., & Oliphant, B. (2020). Family status discrimination: Caregiving and the prima facie case. *Osgoode Hall Law Journal, 56*(3), 564–605. https://doi.org/10.60082/2817-5069.3567

Waddell, C., Schwartz, C., & Andres, C. (2018). Making children's mental health a public policy priority: For the one and the many. *Public Health Ethics, 11*(2), 191–200. https://doi.org/10.1093/phe/phx018

Work Life Law (2025). Laws protecting family caregivers at work. https://worklifelaw.org/wp-content/uploads/State-Local-FRD-Law-List.pdf

9

EMERGING TRENDS AND INNOVATIONS

Families raising children with mental health disabilities are navigating a rapidly shifting, and often uneven, landscape of services, workplace practices, and policy responses. Earlier chapters in this volume have documented persistent gaps in mental health care, employment protections, and family support, as well as the structural inequities that shape how families experience and respond to these gaps. This chapter turns attention to emerging trends and innovations that have begun to challenge some of these longstanding limitations. Rather than focusing on novelty or technological advancement alone, the emphasis here is on changes in how responsibility for care is conceptualized and distributed across systems.

A central argument of this chapter is that innovation for families of children with mental health disabilities is most meaningful when it operates at the level of environments rather than individuals. For many families, particularly those managing episodic and unpredictable care needs, crisis-driven models that rely on individual coping, disclosure, or self-advocacy have proven insufficient and, at times, harmful. In contrast, recent developments in workplace design, organizational practice, family-inclusive mental health care, and social policy suggest a gradual, though incomplete, shift toward recognizing caregiving as a predictable feature of contemporary life rather than an exceptional circumstance. These developments open new possibilities for prevention, employment stability, and family well-being, while also raising important questions about access, equity, and implementation.

The chapter centers workplaces as a critical, yet often underexamined, site of intervention for supporting families raising children with mental health disabilities. It examines emerging organizational strategies, including healthy work design frameworks, family-supportive supervisory practices, human resource professional training, caregiver employee resource groups, and employer-sponsored care navigation, as mechanisms that reshape the conditions under which families manage

DOI: 10.4324/9781003532668-9

care and employment. These workplace innovations are situated alongside family-inclusive mental health interventions and evolving policy frameworks that function as enabling or constraining scaffolds for support. Throughout, the chapter applies a person-in-environment and disability justice lens to assess not only what is changing, but for whom, under what conditions, and with what implications for social work practice, education, and advocacy.

Part 1: Workplace Interventions

For much of the past several decades, the workplace has been positioned primarily as a source of strain for parents raising children with mental health disabilities rather than as a potential site of support. A substantial body of research has documented work–family conflict, stigma, job insecurity, and the risks associated with disclosure and accommodation requests for caregivers managing children's mental health needs (Stewart et al., 2025; Stewart & Charles, 2022; Williams, 2006). While this scholarship has been critical in naming harm and inequity, it has also tended to frame workplaces as relatively fixed environments, leaving parents to navigate risk through individual coping, disclosure, or exit from the labor force.

Recently, this framing has begun to shift. The COVID-19 pandemic, labor market disruptions, and growing attention to worker mental health have accelerated recognition of work as a social determinant of health and family well-being (Hammer et al., 2024; Kniffin et al., 2021; Surgeon General of the United States, 2022). At the same time, advances in organizational psychology and population-level data on caregiving have challenged the assumption that care is exceptional or incompatible with productivity. Instead, caregiving is increasingly understood as a predictable feature of contemporary work lives, affecting workers across occupations, income levels, and family structures (AARP & National Alliance for Caregiving, 2025; Kossek et al., 2023). This shift has important implications for families raising children with mental health disabilities. When caregiving is treated as predictable rather than exceptional, responsibility for managing work–care conflict moves from individual employees toward organizational systems, managerial practices, and employment policies. From a social work perspective, this reframing opens new terrain for preventive, person-in-environment intervention that centers social justice and equity by examining how caregiver strain and employment instability are produced through intersecting systems of power, discrimination, and exclusion. Attending to work design, organizational norms, and policy structures allows social workers to identify how race, gender, disability, class, and immigration status shape differential exposure to risk and unequal access to flexibility, protection, and support. This shifts practice away from expectations of individual adaptation and resilience and toward equity-oriented interventions that challenge structurally embedded disadvantage and advance more inclusive conditions for families navigating mental health-related caregiving.

Work Redesign Frameworks: The Case for Healthy Work Design

One prominent example of this shift is the growing application of work redesign frameworks that explicitly link job structure and organizational practice to health outcomes. In the United States, the Total Worker Health© (TWH) framework developed by the National Institute for Occupational Safety and Health positions work organization, supervisory practices, and employment policies as central determinants of worker health and well-being (National Institute for Occupational Health and Safety [NIOSH], 2016, 2024). TWH integrates worker safety, health protection, and well-being promotion through systems-level actions, emphasizing leadership commitment, supportive policies, work design, worker engagement, and systems integration. As illustrated in the Total Worker Health hierarchy of controls (see Figure 9.1), interventions that eliminate or redesign harmful conditions are more effective than those that rely on individual behavior change or personal protective strategies (NIOSH, 2016).

For parents raising children with mental health disabilities, TWH offers a useful analytic and practical framework because it directs attention away from individual resilience and toward the design of work itself. Rather than asking how parents can better manage unpredictable caregiving demands within rigid employment structures, TWH asks how work can be designed to reduce exposure to chronic stressors, increase predictability and control, and support health across the workforce. These

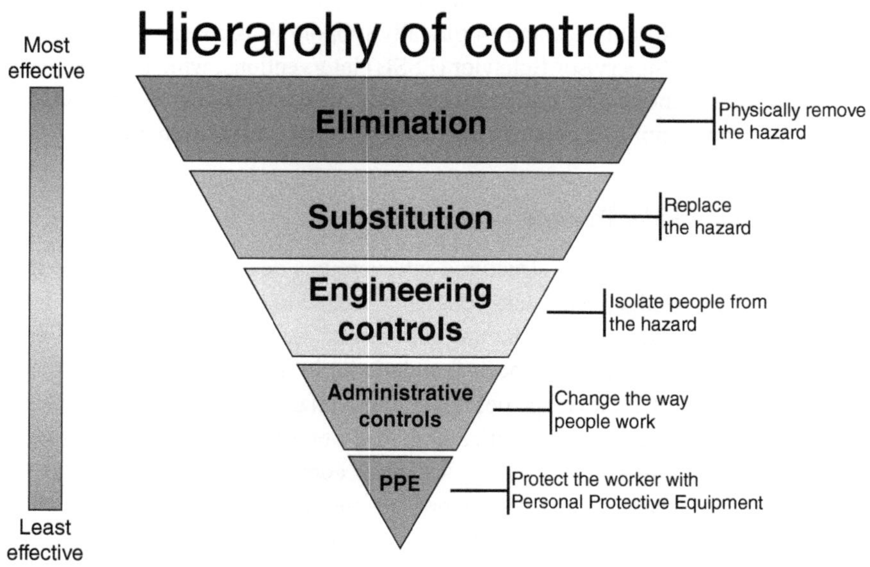

FIGURE 9.1 Total Worker Health Hierarchy of Controls

Source: National Institute for Occupational Safety and Health (NIOSH), Fundamentals of Total Worker Health® approaches: Essential elements for advancing worker safety, health, and well-being (2016).

principles are particularly salient for families managing episodic crises, psychiatric hospitalization, school exclusion, or fluctuating care needs, where rigid schedules and punitive attendance policies can quickly translate into job loss or downward mobility. At the same time, access to healthy work design remains uneven. TWH-informed practices are more common in larger organizations and among higher-wage workers, raising important questions about equity, implementation, and the distribution of benefits. These disparities underscore the importance of examining not only which innovations exist, but who can realistically access them and under what conditions.

The sections that follow examine workplace-based interventions that reflect this broader shift toward organizational responsibility. Rather than focusing on individual accommodations alone, these interventions operate at multiple levels of the work environment, including supervision, human resource practice, organizational culture, and benefit design.

Workplace-Based Interventions

Workplace-based interventions aimed at supporting employees with caregiving responsibilities have increasingly moved away from individualized accommodations toward organizational-level strategies that seek to change how work is designed, managed, and governed (Kossek et al., 2014, 2023). These approaches recognize that caregiving-related strain is not simply a function of individual need, but of how policies are interpreted, how supervisors exercise discretion, and how organizational norms shape access to flexibility and support.

One of the most established and empirically supported approaches in this area is Family-Supportive Supervisor Behavior (FSSB) interventions, which treat supervisory behavior as a modifiable mechanism through which work–family conflict, caregiver strain, and employee mental health may be addressed (Hammer et al., 2024).

Supervisor and Leader Training

Supervisory training refers to structured interventions designed to equip supervisors with the knowledge, skills, and behaviors needed to support employees' work and nonwork demands in ways that promote health, safety, and well-being. Leslie Hammer's body of research has been foundational in demonstrating that supervisors function as a critical leverage point within organizations because they translate formal policies into everyday practice and shape employees' psychosocial work environments (Hammer et al., 2011). A central contribution of this work is the development and testing of family-supportive supervisor behaviors (FSSB), which emphasize emotional support, instrumental support, role modeling, and creative work–family management. Randomized controlled trials show that training supervisors in these behaviors leads to improvements in job satisfaction, reductions in work–family conflict, lower psychological distress, improved sleep, and better safety outcomes among employees (Hammer et al., 2011, 2024). Importantly, these effects are achieved without requiring employees to disclose personal circumstances or individually negotiate accommodations.

Within the Total Worker Health framework, supervisory training functions as an organizational-level intervention rather than an individual behavior change strategy. By altering how supervisors structure work, respond to caregiving needs, and communicate expectations, training reshapes the social context of work in ways that produce sustained health benefits (Hammer et al., 2011). Supportive supervisory behaviors reduce chronic stressors such as time pressure, role conflict, and fear of negative consequences for requesting support, all of which are strongly associated with psychological distress and longer-term health risks (Hammer et al., 2024). Supportive supervision also increases employees' perceived control and predictability, which are core determinants of occupational health. When flexibility is legitimate and responses to caregiving needs are consistent rather than punitive, employees experience greater autonomy over how and when work is completed. This increased sense of control buffers physiological stress responses and reduces anticipatory stress, supporting better mental health and recovery (Hammer & Sauter, 2013). Over time, embedding support-seeking and flexibility into everyday management practices helps normalize caregiving and reduces stigma, particularly for workers managing invisible or episodic needs (Hammer et al., 2024).

Implications for Social Work Practice

The person-in-environment model has long guided social work practice by situating individual distress within broader environmental contexts. The TWH hierarchy of controls extends this logic by ranking intervention targets according to their capacity to reduce harm, directing attention first to upstream conditions that shape exposure to risk. When used together, these frameworks prompt a shift in practice questions, from how parents are coping to how work, school, and service environments are producing or amplifying crisis. Applying the hierarchy of controls alongside the person-in-environment model helps clarify the limits of individual-level interventions when employment instability is driven by rigid schedules, inflexible leave policies, or discretionary supervisory practices. It also provides a shared language for engaging employers, policymakers, and allied professionals in conversations about prevention and systems redesign.

During periods of acute or recurring crisis, such as psychiatric hospitalization or school disruption, social workers can use the hierarchy of controls as a *planning and analytic tool* rather than as a direct mechanism for change. In community practice settings, including mental health clinics, schools, and family service organizations, the hierarchy of controls can provide social work practitioners with a structured way to identify where environmental risk is being produced for parents and to clarify which levels of intervention are most likely to reduce harm over time. At the macro and mezzo levels, this work often takes the form of documentation, pattern recognition, and strategic advocacy, rather than immediate policy change. For example, when multiple families experience job loss or disciplinary action during predictable periods of child mental health crisis, social workers are well positioned to identify these outcomes as structurally produced rather than individually driven. Through case documentation, aggregate reporting, and collaboration with supervisors, administrators, or community partners, social workers can surface how policies such as zero-tolerance attendance rules, inflexible scheduling, or mandatory in-person work function as upstream risk factors for employment instability.

Social workers might also serve an intermediary role by translating family experiences into organizational or policy-relevant language. This could include writing supporting letters, participating in school or hospital discharge planning with attention to caregiver employment risks, consulting with employer-based programs or legal advocacy organizations, or connecting families to worker advocacy and civil rights resources. While these actions do not eliminate harmful policies, they can reduce exposure to risk, strengthen families' negotiating positions, and contribute to longer-term organizational or policy change. At the individual level, social workers continue to provide emotional support, care navigation, and decision support, while explicitly naming the limits of individual coping strategies in the face of rigid systems. Framing intervention in this way helps avoid locating responsibility solely with parents and instead situates employment disruption as a predictable consequence of environmental design. Integrating the TWH hierarchy of controls into person-in-environment informed practice legitimizes work with employers and organizations as core social work practice rather than ancillary advocacy. It also reframes employment stability as an outcome produced by supportive systems rather than individual endurance.

Human Resource Professional Training

In parallel with supervisory interventions, a smaller but growing body of work has focused on human resource (HR) professionals as an intervention population. HR professionals play a central role in shaping policy interpretation, disclosure processes, and access to formal flexibility and benefits, yet have historically received little training related to caregiving for children with disabilities or mental health needs (Stewart et al., 2022).

BOX 9.1 TARGETED HR DIVERSITY TRAINING AS AN ORGANIZATIONAL-LEVEL INTERVENTION

Overview

Parents of children with mental health disabilities often face workplace barriers not because policies are absent, but because they are inconsistently interpreted and applied. Human resource (HR) professionals play a key gatekeeping role in shaping access to flexibility, accommodations, leave, and disclosure processes. This case study describes a targeted diversity training intervention developed by Stewart et al. (2022) to address this implementation gap by reframing caregiving for children with disabilities as a workplace inclusion issue rather than an individual employee problem.

Intervention Design

The intervention was evaluated with 54 HR professionals recruited from U.S. offices of an international accounting firm (KPMG). Participants held roles involving employee relations, policy interpretation, or accommodation decision-making. Recruitment prioritized implementation relevance over representativeness.

The training focused on:

- *Work–family realities of caregiving for children with disabilities, including mental health disabilities*
- *Relevant legal and policy frameworks*
- *Organizational consequences of unsupported caregiving, such as turnover and inequitable treatment*

The training emphasized proactive, preventive responses rather than compliance-only approaches and included guided exercises on responding to employee disclosures.

Framing within the Total Worker Health Hierarchy of Controls

Viewed through the Total Worker Health© hierarchy of controls, the intervention functions as an organizational-level control rather than an individual coping strategy (NIOSH, 2016). While caregiving demands cannot be eliminated, the training targets avoidable organizational harms by substituting rigid or discretionary decision-making with more consistent, informed practices.

At the administrative control level, the training reshaped how HR professionals interpret policies and advise managers. Post-training, participants showed greater willingness to proactively consider flexible work arrangements, recognize caregiving as ongoing rather than episodic, and normalize flexibility as a workforce sustainability strategy. These shifts reduce reliance on parental self-advocacy and repeated disclosure of sensitive information.

Key Findings and Implications

Evaluation findings indicated improvements in HR professionals' knowledge of disability-related caregiving, perceived competence in responding to employee needs, and endorsement of flexible workplace practices. Importantly, the intervention reduced narrow compliance-based responses and encouraged broader, equity-oriented interpretations of policy.

For parents of children with mental health disabilities, this case illustrates how modest, scalable organizational interventions can reduce invisible labor and exposure to risk. By intervening upstream, at the level of HR knowledge and norms, the training supports employment continuity without requiring new legislation or major financial investment.

Further Reading

Stewart, L. M., Rosenzweig, J. M., Malsch Tamarkin, A. M., & Brennan, E. M. (2022). Expanding workplace inclusion of employees who are parents of children with disabilities through diversity training. Healthcare, 10(23), 361. https://doi.org/10.3390/healthcare10122361

Interventions targeting HR professionals aim to increase awareness of caregiving-related stigma, improve understanding of mental health–related caregiving needs, and promote more consistent and equitable responses to caregiver disclosures and requests (Stewart et al., 2022). Rather than eliminating the need for individual employees to engage with HR, these interventions seek to reduce discretionary variability and create conditions of greater psychological safety for parents navigating formal workplace processes. By strengthening HR professionals' understanding of how caregiving for a child with a disability differs from caregiving for typically developing children, such approaches aim to improve organizational responses without increasing the burden on individual caregivers.

Worker-Focused Interventions

Alongside interventions targeting supervisors and HR professionals, an emerging literature has examined worker-focused interventions designed to support caregivers in navigating disclosure and access to workplace support within existing organizational conditions. Research consistently shows that disclosure is a conditional and context-dependent strategy. While disclosure can enable access to flexibility and leave, it also exposes caregivers to stigma, reduced advancement opportunities, and job insecurity, particularly when care needs are unpredictable or poorly understood (AARP & National Alliance for Caregiving, 2025; Stewart & Charles, 2022).

Interventions such as caregiver-focused decision aids and coaching programs aim to support more informed and strategic disclosure decision-making. Decision aids grounded in shared decision-making frameworks help caregivers clarify values, weigh risks and benefits, and identify appropriate timing and recipients of disclosure, with emerging evidence of reduced decisional conflict and increased confidence (Stacey et al., 2017; Stewart et al., 2025). Coaching and training interventions may improve perceived preparedness and self-efficacy, but their effectiveness remains contingent on upstream workplace conditions.

BOX 9.2 WORKER-FOCUSED DISCLOSURE DECISION SUPPORT: THE MYCHOICE WORKPLACE DISCLOSURE DECISION AID

Overview

One emerging worker-focused intervention for parents of children with mental health disabilities is the MyChoice Workplace Disclosure Decision Aid (Stewart et al., under review). Developed through a NIOSH-funded study, MyChoice supports parents facing high-stakes, preference-sensitive decisions about whether, when, and how to disclose their child's mental health needs in the workplace.

Conceptual Foundation

MyChoice is grounded in the Ottawa Decision Support Framework, an evidence-based model designed to assist individuals navigating complex decisions under conditions of uncertainty, competing values, and risk (O'Connor et al., 1998; Stacey et al., 2017). The framework emphasizes values clarification and decisional support rather than advice-giving or prescriptive guidance.

What the Intervention Supports

Rather than promoting disclosure as inherently beneficial, MyChoice centers psychological safety and recognizes that disclosure decisions are shaped by supervisory practices, organizational culture, job security, and stigma related to both mental health and caregiving (Stewart et al., under review). The tool helps parents:

- *Clarify values related to privacy, employment stability, and access to support*
- *Weigh perceived risks and benefits of disclosure in specific workplace contexts*
- *Anticipate likely organizational responses*
- *Identify available formal and informal supports*

Preferences for sharing sensitive information are treated as contextual and experience-based, allowing parents to weigh competing priorities rather than move toward a predetermined outcome (Stewart et al., under review).

Emerging Evidence

Results from a national pilot study showed significant reductions in decisional conflict among parents using MyChoice (Stewart et al., under review). This finding is notable given the established association between decisional conflict and heightened stress, anxiety, and psychological distress in uncertain contexts (O'Connor, 1995; Stacey et al., 2017).

Limits and System Dependence

Within a Total Worker Health perspective, MyChoice functions as a bounded, preventive intervention by reducing cognitive and emotional load at a critical decision point and by making visible the workplace conditions that shape psychological safety (NIOSH, 2016, 2024). However, the tool does not alter organizational policies, supervisory practices, or legal protections. Its effectiveness depends on upstream workplace conditions and should be understood as complementary to, rather than a substitute for, organizational- and policy-level interventions that reduce reliance on individual disclosure as the primary pathway to support.

Overall, the evidence suggests that worker-focused interventions can support individual decision-making but cannot mitigate structural risk in the absence of supportive supervisors, organizational policies, and workplace cultures.

Part 2: Family Interventions

As already discussed in Chapter 6, family support and inclusion is often still missing or limited in mental health interventions, despite its proven positive impact on recovery and treatment outcomes (British Psychological Society, 2021; Kopelovich et al., 2021). According to a 2017 report, only about 2% of families in the U.S. received family support interventions (Interdepartmental Serious Mental Illness Coordinating Committee, 2017 as cited by Kopelovich et al., 2021). The following section will introduce some innovative approaches to integrating family support in mental health services. This is not an exhaustive list, but a snapshot of interventions and strategies that hopefully provides initial ideas and ignites curiosity to go deeper and look for strategies to be implemented in one's own context.

In 2021, the *British Psychological Society Division of Clinical Psychology and the faculty of Complex Mental Health and Psychosis* developed recommendations for practitioners working with families dealing with psychosis. They point out that family interventions and family support have been identified as crucial but that in practice interventions often still fall short and more likely focus on the individual with a diagnosis excluding the individual's larger social support network. In summary, these recommendations stress the importance of family-inclusive practices not just to support family members who are also impacted by a mental health diagnosis, but to improve the health and well-being of the individual with a mental health disability, since relapse and rehospitalization rates are lower for individuals whose families were included in interventions.

At the heart of their model is the recommendation that any agency or individual provider should center their practice on the premise of a family-friendly/sensitive and family-inclusive approach (see Figure 9.2).

The acknowledgement of the importance of family support and the commitment to including family members should infuse all practice steps and agency policies. It is important to mention in this context that family is defined broadly and individually. Service users should define who family is for them including people in their social networks that provide social, emotional, and/or instrumental support and care. A family-sensitive and inclusive approach also moves away from defining families or family members and behaviors as problematic or dysfunctional but understands behaviors as coping strategies within an existing context of available

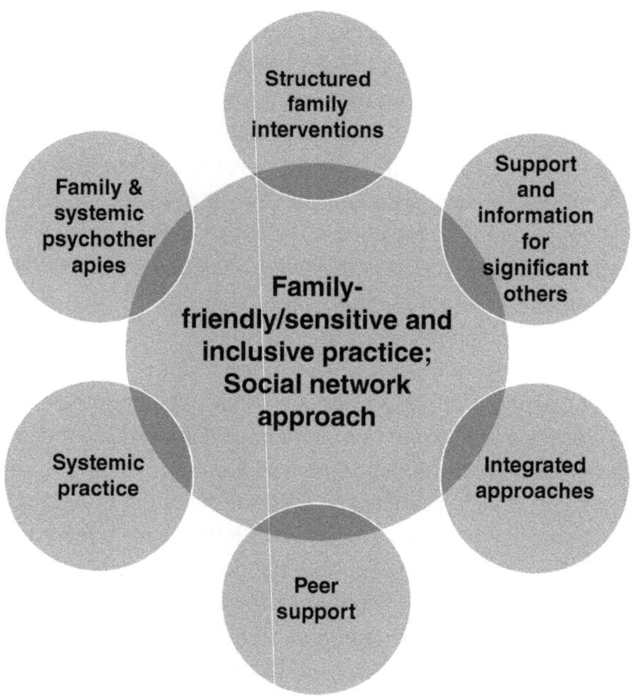

FIGURE 9.2 Model for Family-inclusive Practice

Source: Figure is based on 2021 British Psychological Society Division of Clinical Psychology and the faculty of Complex Mental Health and Psychosis recommendations

resources and skills. Therapeutic or psycho-educational interventions can help families to develop additional coping strategies and support a transition from survival to thriving, adaptation, and resilience. Based on this centering of families or social networks, providers and agencies might offer different specific interventions, such as systemic family or behavioral family therapy, peer support programs or psychoeducational groups.

Open Dialogue is one intervention approach, which could be used within this framework. It has been developed in the 1980s in Finland (Seikkula, 2003) and is therefore technically not an emerging intervention, but it is more recent that it has been adopted in the United States. In this approach, family members are active participants and part of the treatment planning and implementation process. Families are not relegated to separate family therapy sessions, but integral to the whole treatment process. Family is also conceptualized broadly, and anyone of relevance in the service user's social network can be part of the ongoing treatment meetings. Dialogue itself and not family change is the intervention goal and intervention tool. Through open dialogue individuals can normalize their experience and strengthen their coping skills. Open dialogue is practiced in team meetings that include all professionals involved in the treatment in addition to the service users and their social network members.

Psychosis REACH, which stands for Recovery by Enabling Adult Carers at Home, is a family intervention developed by faculty at the University of Washington in the United States. It offers a day-long workshop to family members of individuals with a psychosis diagnosis. The training includes three components. First family members receive recovery-oriented psychoeducation about the condition to address fears and myths about the diagnosis and about standards of care to also support them in advocacy for their family members. The component of caregiver self-care includes information about standard approaches to self-care such as managing boundaries or nutrition but also applies cognitive behavioral therapy principles to the caregiving experience. Finally, family members learn cognitive behavioral therapy skills to strengthen family interactions. The project also trained family ambassadors, who are more experienced family members who support family members newly receiving the REACH training. Family ambassadors can offer ongoing support for skill development after the initial workshop. Initial evaluation of the intervention found a reduction in depression and anxiety scores and an increase in CBT-informed caregiving skills. These effects persisted in a 4-month follow-up (Kopelovich et al., 2021). This would be another example for a family inclusive intervention approach.

Additionally, there are changes and innovations to the delivery model of interventions. This does not only include online or text-based therapy, but also AI-based mental health apps for children (Yang et al., 2025) and caregivers (Premanandan et al., 2024). These apps are no replacement for therapeutic interventions but could augment the support system and increase access. As became obvious during the pandemic, access to any digital or online form of support also requires the availability of technology, the ability to navigate the technology, and internet access, which could further exacerbate access barriers.

Part 3: Social and Workplace Policies

As discussed in Chapter 7, during the COVID-19 pandemic, the U.S. Congress passed emergency requirements for paid sick leave and paid Family Medical Leave as well as an expansion of the child tax credit. Unfortunately, these emergency provisions were not extended, despite their positive impact. As we have seen in Chapter 8 looking at other countries, these provisions can hardly be considered innovative in the global context. It still seems important to mention these policy developments in this chapter on emerging trends, since they demonstrate the potential for change and expansion of family-supportive policies. The growing number of states with state programs for paid family and medical leave or paid sick leave laws are another set of examples that should keep social work energized in its political advocacy efforts.

We would also like to mention the 2016 21st Century Cures Act as another example of innovative legislation that has had a positive impact on the availability of mental health care in the United States. This legislation includes sections on supporting individuals and families in mental health crises, on expanding the mental health care workforce, and on increasing mental health and substance use treatment access, including funding to states for increasing mental health care. This legislation required the formation of the Interdepartmental Serious Mental Illness Coordinating Committee, which published a report on the state of mental health and substance use care in the United States in 2017 and 2022, reporting, for example, that only 2% of families receive family support. Another result of this collaboration was the development of the National Guidelines for Behavioral Health Crisis Care Best Practice Toolkit, which stipulated the three core aspects of an adequate crisis response as a 24/7 crisis line, mobile crisis teams, and facilities for crisis stabilizations (Substance Abuse and Mental Health Services Administration, 2020). In 2022, the United States also transitioned to the 3-digit crisis hotline number 988, mimicking the 911 emergency phone number, enabling easier access to this life-saving service. The 2022 Interdepartmental Serious Mental Illness Coordinating Committee report also shared that 96% of states offered a 24-hour crisis hotline, 94% funded mobile crisis teams, and 92% provided state funding for stabilization facilities (Interdepartmental Serious Mental Illness Coordinating Committee, 2022). The 2022 Mental Health Matters Act is another example of the growing recognition of the need for mental health care, specifically increasing access to school-based mental health care (House Committee on Education and Labor, n.d.)

Right-to-Request and Related Workplace Initiatives

An emerging trend in workplace policy which signals shifting recognition of caregiving as a workforce reality is the expansion of right-to-request flexible working legislation. Right-to-request laws provide employees with a statutory entitlement to formally request changes to their working arrangements, such as hours, schedules, or work location, and require employers to consider those requests through a defined process, even when approval is not guaranteed (Advisory, Conciliation and Arbitration Service [Acas], n.d.; International Labour Organization [ILO], 2022). Internationally, right-to-request frameworks have been implemented across multiple jurisdictions. In the United Kingdom, the right to request flexible working was initially introduced for parents and carers and later expanded to all employees, with recent reforms strengthening employer obligations and extending eligibility to day-one employment (UK Department for Business and Trade, n.d.). At the European level, the EU Work–Life Balance Directive requires member states to provide parents and carers with the right to request flexible working arrangements, reflecting broader recognition of care as a structural feature of employment rather than an exception (European Commission, 2019). Similar provisions exist in Australia under the Fair Work Act, which allows carers to request flexibility that may only be refused on reasonable business grounds (Fair Work Ombudsman, n.d.).

BOX 9.3 THE EU WORK–LIFE BALANCE DIRECTIVE: IMPLICATIONS FOR PARENTS OF CHILDREN WITH MENTAL HEALTH DISABILITIES

Overview

The EU Work–Life Balance Directive (Directive 2019/1158) represents a significant shift in work–family policy by reframing flexible working as a core mechanism for reconciling paid work and caregiving across the life course, rather than as a narrow accommodation tied to parental leave transitions (European Union, 2019). Introduced in 2019, the Directive strengthens procedural rights while preserving employer discretion, with particular relevance for parents of children with disabilities.

Expanded Recognition of Caregiving

A central innovation of the Directive is its expansion of who holds the right to request flexible working. In addition to parents of young children, the policy explicitly recognizes "carers" as rights-bearing workers, defined as individuals providing personal care or support to a child, relative, or household member with a serious medical condition (European Union, 2019). This recognition is especially salient for parents of children with mental health disabilities, whose caregiving responsibilities often extend well beyond early childhood and do not align with traditional parental leave periods.

Broader Definitions of Flexible Working

The Directive broadens what counts as flexible working to include remote work, adjusted schedules, reduced hours, and predictable return rights. This expanded definition better reflects the episodic and crisis-driven nature of children's mental health needs, where parents may require short-term or intermittent flexibility rather than extended leave. Importantly, the right to return to the original working arrangement reduces long-term career risk associated with using flexibility (European Union, 2019).

Procedural Rights and Legal Protections

The Directive establishes a procedural, rather than substantive, right to flexible working. Employers are required to consider requests, respond within a reasonable timeframe, and justify refusals or postponements, but are not obligated to grant them (European Union, 2019). While this stops short of guaranteeing access, it creates transparency and accountability and reduces reliance on managerial goodwill alone. The Directive also strengthens protections against discrimination or adverse treatment related to requesting or using flexible work and operates alongside EU equality law, including protections against discrimination by association (Coleman v. Attridge Law, 2008).

Implications for Families

For parents of children with mental health disabilities, the Directive illustrates both the promise and limits of emerging policy approaches. By recognizing caregiving across the life course and formalizing negotiation processes, it reduces some employment risks associated with episodic care. At the same time, its effectiveness depends on national implementation and enforcement, underscoring that procedural rights alone are necessary but insufficient to ensure meaningful support.

Implementation across European Member States, however, reveals uneven protection in practice (Migration Policy Group, 2022). Germany has expanded flexibility within its parental leave system through income-related reforms such as *ElterngeldPlus*, which allow parents to extend benefit duration and combine leave with part-time employment (OECD, 2026). Sweden's parental leave system permits substantial transferability of leave days between parents, with most days transferable under defined conditions and high earnings-related replacement rates that support uptake (Blum et al., 2023; OECD, 2026). In contrast, Belgium and France rely more heavily on flat-rate parental leave benefits, where lower replacement levels may discourage uptake among families experiencing economic strain (Blum et al., 2023; OECD, 2026).

The United States does not have any federal right to request protections. Instead, a patchwork of laws across the country serves to provide some workers with the right to request an adjustment to where and how they work (see Vermont's Flexible Working Arrangement Statute 21 V.S.A. § 309 or the city of San Francisco's Family Friendly Work Ordinance). Evidence on outcomes suggests that right-to-request policies can modestly increase access to reduced or modified working hours and are associated with improvements in well-being for some workers, particularly women with caregiving responsibilities (Chung & van der Horst, 2018; International Labour Organization, 2022; Waddington & Bell, 2021).

Although right-to-request legislation establishes an important procedural framework and reduces sole reliance on managerial discretion, its effectiveness depends on national implementation, enforcement mechanisms, and integration with broader equality and anti-discrimination protections. The United States, by contrast, does not currently provide a federal statutory right to request flexible working arrangements. Right-to-request legislation and related policy initiatives illustrate the ambivalent nature of emerging workplace trends. They reflect growing institutional acknowledgment that caregiving is a predictable feature of contemporary work, yet they stop short of guaranteeing meaningful support. For families navigating the uncertainty described throughout this book, these developments represent important possibilities that can enhance psychological safety and employment sustainability, but only when paired with supportive organizational cultures, trained supervisors, and policy scaffolding that recognizes the realities of disability-related caregiving.

Part 4: Summary and Key Points

This chapter has examined a set of emerging trends and innovations across workplaces, family-centered mental health practice, technology, and social and workplace policy. Although these developments vary in form and scope, they share a common orientation toward shifting responsibility away from individual families and toward the environments in which care, employment, and service access are negotiated. In contrast to crisis-driven and deficit-oriented approaches, the innovations reviewed here emphasize prevention, predictability, and collective responsibility, consistent with person-in-environment and disability justice perspectives (Oliver, 1990; Piepzna-Samarasinha, 2018). Across domains, the most consequential developments are those that reduce families' reliance on individualized and high-risk strategies, including repeated disclosure, ad hoc negotiation, or withdrawal from paid work. In workplace contexts, healthy work design frameworks, family-supportive supervisory practices, HR professional training, caregiver employee resource groups, and employer-sponsored care navigation illustrate how flexibility and coordination can be embedded within organizational systems rather than contingent on individual advocacy or managerial goodwill (AARP, 2024; Hammer et al., 2016; Kossek et al., 2014). In mental health service settings, family-inclusive and network-based interventions similarly redistribute responsibility by positioning families and social networks as integral to care, rather than as optional or ancillary supports (British Psychological Society, 2021; Kopelovich et al., 2021).

The chapter highlights important limitations. Access to workplace innovations remains uneven, with benefits disproportionately concentrated among higher-wage workers and larger employers (AARP & National Alliance for Caregiving, 2025; National Academies of Sciences, Engineering, and Medicine, 2023). Digital and AI-enabled supports depend on access to technology and digital literacy and may exacerbate existing inequities if implemented without attention to access and context (Premanandan et al., 2024; Yang et al., 2025). Similarly, procedural policy protections, such as right-to-request frameworks, often fail to translate into substantive change in everyday practice, particularly for families managing episodic and unpredictable care needs (Waddington & Bell, 2021). Without explicit attention to implementation and equity, emerging innovations risk reproducing existing stratifications rather than mitigating them. The evidence reviewed in this chapter suggests that employment stability, caregiver well-being, and family mental health are most effectively supported when interventions operate upstream and are reinforced across systems. This synthesis reinforces the chapter's central argument: sustained support for parents of children with mental health disabilities depends less on individual adaptation and resilience and more on how work, care, and social protection are collectively organized (Voydanoff, 2005; World Health Organization & International Labour Organization, 2022).

Part 5: Implications for Social Work Practice

The trends discussed in this chapter have several implications for social work practice, especially for practitioners working in community-based settings such as mental health clinics, schools, and family service organizations. These implications do not presume that frontline social workers have direct authority to alter workplace policies or labor regulations. Rather, they point to shifts in assessment, framing, and intervention priorities that align with person-in-environment and prevention-oriented practice.

First, social work practice with families raising children with mental health disabilities should routinely attend to employment conditions as a core dimension of family well-being. Work schedules, supervisory relationships, access to flexibility, and benefit structures shape families' capacity to manage care and should be considered alongside clinical, educational, and service needs (Kossek et al., 2023; Voydanoff, 2005). Interventions that support parents with disclosure decisions, care navigation, or crisis planning may be appropriate, but these strategies should be framed as bounded supports rather than as primary solutions to structurally produced risk (Stacey et al., 2017; Stewart et al., 2022).

Second, social workers occupy an important intermediary position in documenting and interpreting patterns of harm across cases. Through case records, supervision, program evaluation, and collaboration with administrators and community partners, social workers can identify how rigid workplace practices, school policies, or service system constraints predictably contribute to employment disruption and caregiver strain. Over time, this documentation can inform organizational consultation, cross-sector partnerships, and policy advocacy, even when individual practitioners lack formal decision-making authority (National Academies of Sciences, Engineering, and Medicine, 2023; Williams, 2006).

Third, the chapter underscores the importance of recognizing employer-facing, organizational, and policy-oriented activities as legitimate forms of social work practice. Consultation with organizations, participation in interdisciplinary initiatives, collaboration with legal and worker advocacy groups, and engagement in policy development are consistent with social work's ethical commitments and theoretical foundations. These activities extend practice beyond individual service provision toward shaping the societal and environmental conditions that influence family stability and well-being (Oliver, 1990; Soldatic & Chapman, 2010).

Finally, the limits of existing employment-based systems highlight the need for continued examination of alternative approaches to economic security and care. Reliance on continuous full-time employment as the primary pathway to income, benefits, and stability remains poorly aligned with the realities of disability-related caregiving. Emerging discussions of universal basic income, mutual aid, and care as interdependence rather than dependency offer important directions for future social work research, teaching, and advocacy (Nadasen, 2023; Piepzna-Samarasinha, 2018). Disability justice scholarship is particularly relevant in this regard, as it foregrounds collective responsibility and challenges individualizing narratives of resilience.

Together, these implications position social work as a field with a central role in interpreting, translating, and evaluating emerging innovations. By maintaining sustained attention to environments, equity, and prevention, social work can contribute to ensuring that innovation supports stability and dignity for families raising children with mental health disabilities, rather than shifting additional risk onto those already navigating structural constraint.

Part 6: Application for Social Work Education

ACTIVITY: MAPPING ENVIRONMENTAL RISK AND BOUNDED INTERVENTION

Purpose

Competency 2: Advance Human Rights and Social, Racial, Economic, and Environmental Justice

Competency 3: Engage Anti-Racism, Diversity, Equity, and Inclusion (ADEI) in Practice

Competency 5: Engage in Policy Practice

Competency 7: Assess Individuals, Families, Groups, Organizations, and Communities

This exercise applies a person-in-environment framework and the Total Worker Health hierarchy of controls to caregiving-related employment risk. The focus is on identifying how environmental conditions shape vulnerability and clarifying what forms of intervention are feasible within community-based social work practice.

Scenario

A parent of a 13-year-old child with a serious mental health condition receives services through a community mental health clinic. Over the past year, the child has experienced repeated crises, including emergency department visits and school exclusion. The parent works full time in a position with limited schedule control. Although flexible work policies exist, access depends on supervisory discretion. The parent has not disclosed their child's mental health needs and has received attendance warnings.

Step 1: Identify Environmental Risk

Identify key environmental conditions contributing to employment risk (for example, workplace practices, service system demands, or policy gaps).

Prompt: Which risks are predictable given the structure of work and care, rather than individual choices?

Step 2: Apply the Hierarchy of Controls

Using the Total Worker Health hierarchy, identify:

- **Upstream conditions producing avoidable harm**
- **Organizational practices** that could reduce risk without requiring disclosure
- **Individual supports and their limits**

Prompt: Which actions are within the social worker's direct role, and which require indirect strategies such as documentation, consultation, or referral?

Step 3: Bounded Intervention Planning

Develop a brief plan that includes:

- **One individual-level support**
- One action aimed at environmental conditions
- One limitation that cannot be addressed without broader change

Reflection

How does this exercise reframe disclosure and resilience? How does naming limits of intervention shift responsibility away from the parent and toward systems?

Resource List

Work, care, and organizational contexts

Kossek, E. E., & Lee, K. H. (2023). *Managing work–life boundaries in organizations*. Routledge.

A foundational text on organizational systems, supervisory practices, and flexibility, useful for understanding how work design shapes caregiver experiences beyond individual accommodation.

Williams, J. C. (2010). *Reshaping the work–family debate: Why men and class matter*. Harvard University Press.

A critical examination of workplace norms, stigma, and inequality that remains influential in work–family and caregiving scholarship.

Family inclusion, mental health, and disability

British Psychological Society. (2021). *Family interventions in psychosis: Guidelines for psychologists and practitioners supporting families and social networks*.

A practice-oriented guide that foregrounds family inclusion and social networks as central to effective mental health care.

Hoagwood, K. E., Jensen, P. S., Acri, M. C., Olin, S. S., & Burton, G. (2017). *Responding to the needs of children with serious emotional disturbance*. Springer.

Offers a systems and family-centered perspective on child mental health services, emphasizing coordination and caregiver support.

Oliver, M. (1990). *The politics of disablement*. Macmillan.

A foundational text for understanding disability as socially produced, informing the chapter's emphasis on environmental rather than individual responsibility.

Policy, care, and social protection

Nadasen, P. (2023). *Care: The highest stage of capitalism*. Haymarket Books.

A contemporary political economy analysis of care that challenges individualized models of responsibility and aligns with broader debates on care, work, and social protection.

International Labour Organization. (2022). *Care at work: Investing in care leave and flexible working arrangements*. ILO.

Provides comparative policy analysis relevant to right-to-request frameworks and caregiving across the life course.

Piepzna-Samarasinha, L. L. (2018). *Care work: Dreaming disability justice*. Arsenal Pulp Press.

A key disability justice text that reframes care as collective, relational, and political, offering an important counterpoint to market-based approaches.

References

21st Century Cures Act (2016). https://www.congress.gov/bill/114th-congress/house-bill/34

AARP. (2024). *Why more employers are investing in caregiver employee resource groups*. AARP. https://www.aarp.org/work/employers/info-2024/caregiver-employee-resource-groups.html

AARP, & National Alliance for Caregiving. (2025). *Caregiving in the United States 2025*. AARP. https://www.aarp.org/pri/topics/ltss/family-caregiving/caregiving-in-the-us-2025/

Advisory, Conciliation and Arbitration Service [Acas] (n.d.). Statutory flexible working requests: The right to request. https://www.acas.org.uk/statutory-flexible-working-requests/the-right-to-request

Blum, S., Dobrotić, I., Kaufman, G., Koslowski, A., & Moss, P. (2023). 19th international review of leave policies and related research 2023. International Network On Leave Policies and Research. https://www.leavenetwork.org/fileadmin/user_upload/k_leavenetwork/annual_reviews/2023/Blum_etal_LPRN_full_report_2023.pdf

British Psychological Society Division (2021). Family interventions in psychosis. Guidelines for psychologists and practitioners supporting families and social networks. https://explore.bps.org.uk/binary/bpsworks/8d5e93f37ef93aa0/6f9b1f52231c12bfd96fd69f80b38e60af29eedac01780db9a8c909e2a85ee4a/rep151_2021.pdf

Chung, H., & van der Horst, M. (2018). Women's employment patterns after childbirth and the perceived access to and use of flexitime and teleworking. *Human Relations*, *71*(1), 47–72. https://doi.org/10.1177/0018726717713828

Court of Justice of the European Union. (2008). *Coleman v. Attridge Law and Steve Law* (Case C-303/06), ECLI:EU:C:2008:415. https://eur-lex.europa.eu/legal-content/EN/TXT/?uri=CELEX:62006CJ0303

European Union. (2019). *Directive (EU) 2019/1158 of the European Parliament and of the Council of 20 June 2019 on work-life balance for parents and carers and repealing Council Directive 2010/18/EU*. Official Journal of the European Union, L 188, 79–93. https://eur-lex.europa.eu/eli/dir/2019/1158/oj

Fair Work Ombudsman (n.d.). Flexibility in the workplace. https://www.fairwork.gov.au/employment-conditions/flexibility-in-the-workplace

Hammer, L. B., Dimoff, J., Mohr, C. D., & Allen, S. J. (2024). A framework for protecting and promoting employee mental health through supervisor supportive behaviors. *Occupational Health Science*, *8*, 243–268. https://doi.org/10.1007/s41542-023-00171-x

Hammer, L. B., Johnson, R. C., Crain, T. L., Bodner, T., Kossek, E. E., Davis, K. D., ... & Berkman, L. (2016). Intervention effects on safety compliance and citizenship behaviors: Evidence from the Work, Family, and Health Study. *Journal of Applied Psychology*, *101*(2), 190.

Hammer, L. B., Kossek, E. E., Anger, W. K., Bodner, T., & Zimmerman, K. L. (2011). Clarifying work–family intervention processes: The roles of work–family conflict and family-supportive supervisor behaviors. *Journal of Applied Psychology*, *96*(1), 134–150. https://doi.org/10.1037/a0020927

Hammer, L. B., & Sauter, S. (2013). Total Worker Health and work–life stress. *Journal of Occupational and Environmental Medicine*, *55*, S25–S29. https://doi.org/10.1097/JOM.0000000000000043

House Committee on Education and Labor (n.d.) Mental Health Matters Act. https://democrats-edworkforce.house.gov/imo/media/doc/mental_health_matters_act_fact_sheet2.pdf

Interdepartmental Serious Mental Illness Coordinating Committee (2022). Advances through collaboration: Federal action for a system that works for all people living with SMI and SED and their families and caregivers. https://www.samhsa.gov/sites/default/files/meeting/documents/ismicc-report-to-congress-04012022.pdf

International Labour Organization. (2022). Care at work: Investing in care leave and flexible working arrangements. ILO. https://www.ilo.org/sites/default/files/wcmsp5/groups/public/@dgreports/@dcomm/documents/publication/wcms_838653.pdf

Kniffin, K. M., Narayanan, J., Anseel, F., Antonakis, J., Ashford, S. P., Bakker, A. B., … Vugt, M. V. (2021). COVID-19 and the workplace: Implications, issues, and insights for future research and action. *American Psychologist*, *76*(1), 63–77. https://doi.org/10.1037/amp0000716

Kopelovich, S. L., Stiles, B., Monroe-DeVita, M., Hardy, K., Hallgren, K., & Turkington, D. (2021). Psychosis REACH: Effects of a brief CBT-informed training for family and caregivers of individuals with psychosis. *Psychiatric Services*, *72*(11), 1254–1260. https://doi.org/10.1176/appi.ps.202000740

Kossek, E. E., Hammer, L. B., Kelly, E. L., & Moen, P. (2014). Designing work, family & health organizational change initiatives. *Organizational Dynamics*, *43*(1), 53–63. https://doi.org/10.1016/j.orgdyn.2013.10.007

Kossek, E. E., Perrigino, M. B., & Lautsch, B. A. (2023). Work-life flexibility policies from a boundary control and implementation perspective: A review and research framework. *Journal of Management*, *49*(6), 2062–2108. https://doi.org/10.1177/01492063221140354

Migration Policy Group. (2022). The EU Work–Life Balance Directive: Implementation and transposition review. https://www.migpolgroup.com/wp-content/uploads/2022/12/2022_GE_TR_WLB-Directive-2-2.pdf

Nadasen, P. (2023). *Care: The highest stage of capitalism*. Haymarket Books.

NIOSH. (2016). *Fundamentals of Total Worker Health® approaches: Essential elements for advancing worker safety, health, and well-being*. U.S. Department of Health and Human Services, Centers for Disease Control and Prevention, National Institute for Occupational Safety and Health. https://www.cdc.gov/niosh/docs/2017-112/

NIOSH. (2021). *Total Worker Health®: Advancing worker safety, health, and well-being*. U.S. Department of Health and Human Services, Centers for Disease Control and Prevention. https://www.cdc.gov/niosh/twh/

O'Connor, A. M., Tugwell, P., Wells, G., Elmslie, T., Jolly, E., & Hollingworth, G. (1998). A decision aid for women considering hormone therapy after menopause: Decision support framework and evaluation. *Patient Education & Counseling*, *33*(3), 267–279.

OECD. (2026). *PF2.1: Parental leave systems*. OECD Family Database. https://webfs.oecd.org/els-com/Family_Database/PF2_1_Parental_leave_systems.pdf

Oliver, M. (1990). *The politics of disablement*. Macmillan.

Piepzna-Samarasinha, L. L. (2018). *Care work: Dreaming disability justice*. Arsenal Pulp Press. http://search.ebscohost.com/login.aspx?direct=true&scope=site&db=nlebk&db=nlabk&AN=1934092

Premanandan, S., Ahmad, A., Cajander, Å., Ågerfalk, P., & van Gemert-Pijnen, L. (2024). Designing and evaluating IT applications for informal caregivers: Scoping review. *Journal of Medical Internet Research*, *26*(3). https://doi.org/10.2196/57393

Seikkula, J. (2003). Open dialogue integrates individual and systemic approaches in serious psychiatric crises. *Smith College Studies in Social Work, 73*(2), 227–245. https://doi.org/10.1080/00377310309517683

Soldatic, K., & Chapman, A. (2010). Surviving the assault? The Australian Disability Discrimination Act in the neoliberal workplace. *Social Policy & Society, 9*(4), 567–578. https://doi.org/10.1080/14742831003603299

Stacey, D., Légaré, F., Lewis, K., Barry, M. J., Bennett, C. L., Eden, K. B., Holmes-Rovner, M., Llewellyn-Thomas, H., Lyddiatt, A., Thomson, R., & Trevena, L. (2017). Decision aids for people facing health treatment or screening decisions. *The Cochrane Database of Systematic Reviews, 4*(4), CD001431. https://doi.org/10.1002/14651858.CD001431.pub5

Stewart, L. M., & Charles, A. (2022). To disclose or conceal? Workplace disability and eldercare-related disclosure decision-making strategies. *Journal of Family Issues, 43*(6), 1536–1554. https://doi.org/10.1177/0192513X211026965

Stewart, L. M., Rosenzweig, J. M., Malsch Tamarkin, A. M., Brennan, E. M., & Lukefahr, J. (2022). Expanding workplace inclusion of employees who are parents of children with disabilities through diversity training. *Healthcare, 10*(12), 2361. https://doi.org/10.3390/healthcare10122361

Stewart, L. M., Sellmaier, C., Cossio, M., & Morales, M. (under review). Pilot of a Workplace Disclosure Decision Aid and Resources for Employed Parents.

Stewart, L. M., Sellmaier, C., Ferrari, M., Lukefahr, J., & Brennan (July, 2025). Navigating Disclosure at Work When Caring for a Child with a Mental Health Condition. Paper presented at the Work Stress and Health conference, July 8-11, Seattle, WA.

Substance Abuse and Mental Health Services Administration (2020). National guidelines for behavioral health crisis care: Best practice toolkit. https://bja.ojp.gov/sites/g/files/xyckuh186/files/media/document/samsha-national-guidelines.pdf

Surgeon General of the United States. (2022). *The U.S. Surgeon General's framework for workplace mental health and well-being*. U.S. Department of Health and Human Services. https://www.hhs.gov/surgeongeneral/priorities/workplace-well-being/index.html

UK Department for Business and Trade (n.d.). Factsheet: Flexible working. https://assets.publishing.service.gov.uk/media/69a6bf1ca2495f2d259f1397/factsheet-flexible-working-feb-2026.pdf

University of Washington (n.d.). Psychosis REACH toolkit. https://www.psychosisreach.org/resources

Voydanoff, P. (2005). Toward a conceptualization of perceived work-family fit and balance: A demands and resources approach. *Journal of Marriage and Family, 67*(4), 822–836. https://doi.org/10.1111/j.1741-3737.2005.00178.x

Waddington, L., & Bell, M. (2021). The right to request flexible working arrangements under the work-life balance directive – A comparative perspective. *European Labour Law Journal, 12*(4), 508–528. https://doi.org/10.1177/20319525211038270

Williams, J. C. (2006). *One sick child away from being fired: When "Opting out" is not an option.* UC Hastings College of the Law.

World Health Organization & International Labour Organization. (2022). *Mental health at work: Policy brief.* World Health Organization. https://www.who.int/publications/i/item/9789240053052

Yang, F., Wei, J., Zhao, X., & An, R. (2025). Artificial Intelligence–based mobile phone apps for child mental health: Comprehensive review and content analysis. *JMIR mHealth and uHealth, 13*, e58597–e58597. https://doi.org/10.2196/58597

10

SUMMARY AND FUTURE DIRECTIONS

Part 1: Uncertainty as a Throughline for Exceptional Caregiving

Research and policy discussions of disability caregiving often conceptualize it as a more intense form of caregiving accompanied by the assumption that uncertainty is a temporary condition, one that can be reduced through better information, earlier intervention, or more efficient coordination of services. This framing is poorly aligned with the lived realities of parents raising children with mental health disabilities. Across family, work, and community contexts, uncertainty is not episodic or anomalous, but a *defining feature* of disability caregiving that persists across developmental stages and institutional settings. Parents routinely make decisions in the absence of stable diagnoses, predictable symptom trajectories, or reliable access to services, while simultaneously navigating systems that privilege clarity, consistency, and linear progress.

As this book has shown, uncertainty is not generated by parents' indecision or lack of planning but is *structurally produced* through the interaction of care demands and the social contexts in which care occurs. Prior work on family caregiving demonstrates that caregiving exists along a continuum, shifting from typical to exceptional as a function of the intensity, typology, and complexity of care demands, as well as the availability of family, workplace, and community resources (Stewart, 2013; Stewart et al., 2018). When children's mental health needs fluctuate or intensify, families move toward the exceptional end of this continuum, where care demands are cyclical, crisis-driven, and often poorly matched to existing institutional supports. These mismatches generate ongoing uncertainty, particularly when systems require specific eligibility forms, advance notice, or the need to formally disclose a child's mental health status in order to access formal and informal support.

DOI: 10.4324/9781003532668-10

Empirical research with employed parents of children with mental health disabilities illustrates how uncertainty becomes embedded in everyday decision-making. Parents frequently engage in disclosure risk assessment as they weigh whether, when, and how to share information about their child's mental health needs at work, knowing that disclosure may be necessary to obtain flexibility but may also expose them to stigma, retaliation, diminished career opportunities, or even termination from employment (Rosenzweig et al., 2011; Stewart et al., 2025). These dynamics position parents as managers of uncertainty, responsible for coordinating care across fragmented systems while protecting both their child's well-being and their family's security by maintaining paid employment.

Viewing uncertainty as the throughline challenges dominant interpretations of parental behavior that frame delayed decisions, selective disclosure, or reliance on informal supports as indicators of poor coping or noncompliance. Consistent with earlier findings, such strategies are more accurately understood as adaptive responses to systems that are ill equipped to accommodate fluctuating and unpredictable care needs (Stewart, 2013; Stewart et al., 2018; Stewart et al., 2025). Parents draw on experiential knowledge, narrow relational networks to navigate changing circumstances often in the form of crisis (Rosenzweig et al., 2008). This labor remains largely invisible within formal support structures in both the workplace and the community.

Recognizing uncertainty as the organizing condition of caregiving clarifies why many existing supports fail to produce meaningful or sustained relief. Supports designed around linear trajectories, stable needs, or one-time accommodations often collapse when children's mental health needs shift or when family circumstances change. By treating uncertainty as a problem to be eliminated rather than a condition to be accommodated, systems transfer the burden of adaptation onto families themselves. Centering uncertainty as a throughline provides a critical foundation for rethinking how support, practice, and policy might better align with the realities faced by parents of children with mental health disabilities.

Part 2: Cross-Domain Patterns in Parent Experiences

As discussed in this book, parents interact with work and community systems, and the exceptional care experience influences and shapes these interactions. Workplace, family, and community systems can provide resources that support the integration of work and family responsibilities, but they can also create demands making integration more difficult. Across the three domains, there are some shared patterns. For example, across systems, parents experience isolation, since their experience does not follow a typical life course trajectory (Stewart et al., 2018). Parents worry about exclusion, stigmatization, and isolation in the workplace if coworkers and supervisors learn about their child's disability. Similarly, they often avoid friends or other social situations to avoid judgment (Sellmaier & Buckingham, 2022). Their experiences with schools or child care might also not match their friends' experiences, creating social isolation. As discussed in Chapter 6, being questioned by service providers about parenting practices and assumptions that these might be responsible for the child's mental health disability or being dismissed for voicing concerns about a child's behaviors and well-being also creates a sense of isolation. Furthermore, standard behavioral health practices might not meet the needs of parents or children with mental health disabilities. Schools and day care centers have to accommodate children with disabilities and have to provide individualized education plans if appropriate, but expulsion rates for disabled children remain elevated, and long-term outcomes such as high school graduation rates, post-secondary education enrollment, and rates of employment are lower than for young adults without disabilities (U.S. Department of Education, Office for Civil Rights [OCR], 2023). Difficulties to provide adequate education also affect parents' ability to maintain employment (Sellmaier et al., 2020). Flexibility available to parents in the workplace is not adequate to meet the needs of parents with exceptional care responsibilities. For example, coworkers and supervisors might accommodate the need for flexibility if a child is occasionally sick, but more regularly occurring crises or longer absences might not be met with the same support. Even if parents have access to paid sick days, they might not be enough to cover needed absences. In addition, accommodations and protections from discrimination available both in the workplace and in educational systems are not sufficient in their reach to allow for full inclusion and community participation (Gray, 2002; Kinnear et al., 2016).

It is also important to highlight that the experience of uncertainty differs across different groups, as discussed in Chapter 4. For example, research has shown that there are differences in levels of caregiver strain across different racial groups with Black families reporting the lowest levels of caregiver strain. Women are also more likely than men to give up employment or reduce work hours to meet care responsibilities. Income determines the quality of health insurance, and families who can pay out of pocket will have better and quicker access to services. Racial minorities also report more unmet mental health needs. Mental health care might not be culturally appropriate, creating access barriers for example for immigrant families. Economic insecurity and experiences of discrimination based on race or sexual orientation add to caregiver strain exacerbating stress due to exceptional care responsibilities.

Part 3: Rethinking Support under Conditions of Uncertainty

Implications for the Workplace

Dominant models of workplace support are built on assumptions that poorly reflect the lived realities of parents caring for children with mental health needs. Traditional approaches presume stable needs, predictable caregiving demands, and a clear separation between work and family domains, leading to support that is often operationalized through discrete policies or time-limited accommodations (Blom et al., 2025). In practice, employees must disclose personal information, articulate specific needs in advance, and demonstrate continued productivity to access these supports (Stewart et al., 2025). For parents navigating fluctuating, episodic, and crisis-driven care demands, these assumptions make formal workplace support inaccessible, limited, or even risky (Stewart & Charles, 2022).

Empirical research on workplace experiences of employed parents of children with disabilities, including mental health conditions, shows that these employees experience heightened work–family conflict and stress, and that workplace supports can moderate this relationship albeit less strongly compared to those caring for young children of typical development and older adults (Stewart, 2013; Stewart et al., 2023). Our national study found that parents providing exceptional care, including for children with disability, report significantly higher levels of both work-to-family and family-to-work conflict and stress, and that workplace support influences these outcomes (Stewart et al., 2023). These findings underscore the need for family-supportive workplace cultures and targeted workplace supports that extend beyond narrowly defined organizational flexibility and health policies.

Our research along with that of others finds when parents choose to disclose their child's mental health status to supervisors or coworkers in the hopes of securing flexibility or understanding, they may face stigma or job insecurity, illustrating how workplace culture and interpersonal dynamics shape whether supports are enabling or punishing. Reframing support under conditions of uncertainty requires moving beyond accommodation-based models to approaches that recognize caregiving as a determinant of worker health and well-being (Stewart et al., under review). Total Worker Health, developed by the National Institute for Occupational Safety and Health, provides an integrated framework for this shift (National Institute for Occupational Safety and Health [NIOSH], 2016). In the Total Worker Health approach, workplace policies, programs, and practices are designed to integrate protection from job-related safety and health hazards with the promotion of overall worker well-being, acknowledging that psychosocial, organizational, and non-work factors interact to shape health outcomes (NIOSH, 2024). Disability caregiving, within this framework is an environmental stressor impacting the health and wellbeing of workers.

From this perspective, support is not limited to the availability of flexible scheduling or leave policies; it includes the conditions under which these options can be safely and equitably used. Supervisor discretion, workload management, and organizational norms regarding responsiveness and performance become central mechanisms that either enable or undermine support. Research on work–life integration more broadly suggests that organizational and supervisor support can reduce work–family conflict, but that merely having formal policies is insufficient if they are not accessible without penalty or stigma (Blom et al., 2025; Geraldes et al., 2024).

This reframing also challenges reliance on individual-level interventions such as resilience training, disability-affiliated workplace parent groups or employee assistance programs as the primary solutions. While such programs can offer short-term relief, they do little to address structural conditions that produce uncertainty and concentrate risk among workers with exceptional caregiving responsibilities. Instead, a Total Worker Health-informed approach calls for organizational interventions that reduce uncertainty at its source, including predictable scheduling, transparent decision-making processes, supportive supervisory practices, and protections against stigma and retaliation (Leso et al., 2024).

Treating uncertainty as a *design parameter* rather than a deviation from "normal" work shifts responsibility away from individual parents to manage competing demands in isolation as "personal factors" and instead focuses efforts toward organizations that create environments capable of absorbing fluctuation without penalizing workers. Aligning workplace support with Total Worker Health principles advances both health protection and equity, recognizing that supporting parents navigating caregiving for children with mental health needs is integral to sustaining a healthy workforce.

Implications for Community

As discussed throughout this book, parents caring for children with mental health disabilities are often abruptly thrown into figuring out and navigating a complex medical system. Families report about the need to educate themselves, to find the right therapies and treatments, to deal with insurance companies for coverage, and to advocate for their children's treatment. This often starts at the diagnostic stage with parents feeling dismissed initially when voicing concerns. Figuring out what and if the child has a mental health need and after the diagnosis figuring out the right next steps, requires that parents navigate uncertainty. This uncertainty relates to concrete aspects such as finding a therapist, but also more vague aspects such as worry about the future. Parents we have interviewed describe navigating this uncertainty often with the help of peers who have more experience navigating this system. Connecting families who receive a mental health diagnosis with peer support should be one strategy to support families in making sense of this new situation. Peer support can help with more concrete challenges such as insurance coverage as well as the potential emotional impact of a mental health diagnosis. Case management or patient navigators could also fill that role.

Similar to navigating the medical system, changes are also required for the educational system. Students might be eligible for Section 504 accommodations or Individualized Education Programs (IEP). This requires an understanding of education law and the rights of students, connecting parents with advocates and non-profit organizations who provide training and information to parents and especially older students on how to navigate the educational system, would be beneficial. Receiving this referral from the diagnosing medical provider could reduce the time parents have to spend on finding these connections themselves.

Services are highly specialized, which can create the siloing of interconnected needs. For example, the psychiatrist who focuses on diagnosis and medication treatment, the therapist who works with the individual child, the family therapist who works with the family, the school psychologist who assesses the child for educational services. Furthermore, medical and educational services are usually not considering the workplace impacts of exceptional care demands, leaving vital economic and social needs unmet. Greater integration across services and an inclusion of work-related needs is required, which would allow for a more holistic approach. Similar to a total worker health approach, this would enable a total family resilience approach, one that parents do not have to cobble together themselves but that is already integrated into the system.

Part 4: Research Directions and Emerging Tools

Despite growing attention to work-family policy and supervisor support, significant gaps remain in understanding how families navigate care, employment, and disclosure decisions over time when a child has mental health needs. Addressing these gaps is essential for developing policies and practices that are equitable, usable, and responsive to diverse family contexts.

Decision-Making within Families

Future research should examine how families make decisions about flexibility, care allocation, and boundary management inside the household. Existing empirical work is extremely limited and largely dated, with only a small number of studies examining intra-family decision making and most drawing on samples that combine mental health needs with other forms of disability. There is a critical need for contemporary research that centers children with mental health needs specifically and that captures how parents, partners, extended family members, and, where appropriate, children themselves negotiate care responsibilities, employment adjustments, and emotional labor.

Longitudinal and Life Course Perspectives

Longitudinal research is particularly needed to understand how care and employment decisions evolve over time. Families rarely make a single, static decision about work and care. Instead, they adjust repeatedly in response to developmental changes, service access, policy environments, and labor market conditions. Existing longitudinal studies are outdated and lack racial, ethnic, and socioeconomic diversity. New longitudinal designs should track families across key transition points, such as diagnosis, school changes, crises, and transitions to adulthood, to assess cumulative impacts on employment trajectories, economic security, health, and well-being. Without this information, we lack understanding of how these transition points affect the health and well-being of families. As a result, interventions will have limited effects on outcomes.

Cultural Contexts and Family Systems

Although a growing body of research examines work–family boundary management and caregiver experiences, relatively little empirical work has focused explicitly on how families from collectivist cultural contexts navigate work–home boundaries in the context of caring for a child with mental health needs. Future studies should explore how cultural norms around shared caregiving, interdependence, and obligation shape disclosure decisions, use of workplace flexibility, and stress distribution within families. Comparative and mixed methods research would strengthen intervention design because it would move the field from assuming a universal caregiving model to identifying how cultural norms shape help-seeking, disclosure, boundary management, and perceptions of employer support particularly when an employee is caring for a child with a mental health disability.

At the workplace level, comparative research could reveal where organizational practices unintentionally privilege individualistic assumptions, such as expectations of autonomous problem solving, private boundary negotiation, or nuclear family caregiving. In collectivist contexts, caregiving may be distributed across extended family networks, yet stigma, honor norms, or concerns about bringing family matters into public space may shape disclosure decisions differently. Mixed methods designs could combine survey data on policy use with qualitative interviews to uncover why employees do or do not access supports. That evidence could guide employers to design interventions that are culturally responsive, such as supervisor training that addresses cultural variation in disclosure norms, flexible leave that accommodates extended family caregiving roles, and protections that explicitly address stigma tied to mental health and family reputation. It could also inform how benefits are communicated, since uptake often depends on whether policies are perceived as socially safe to use.

At the community level, this research could identify how informal support systems interact with formal workplace resources. In collectivist settings, families may rely heavily on kin networks, faith communities, or ethnic associations, which can buffer strain but may also reinforce stigma. Understanding these dynamics would allow community-based organizations to tailor psychoeducation, peer support, and navigation services in ways that complement workplace interventions rather than duplicating or contradicting them. Mixed methods approaches would help identify which families are underutilizing formal services and why, clarifying whether barriers are structural, cultural, or relational.

At the policy level, comparative evidence could expose how labor and disability policy frameworks embed individualistic assumptions, such as placing the burden of accommodation on individual negotiation or requiring formal documentation processes that may be culturally stigmatizing. Cross-national comparisons could show how more collective policy approaches, such as universal caregiver leave, predictable scheduling mandates, or stronger anti-retaliation protections, shift outcomes. Quantitative data could document disparities in policy uptake across cultural groups, while qualitative findings could explain the mechanisms driving those disparities. This would support policy reform aimed at reducing reliance on individual advocacy and increasing structural protections.

Stress, Health, and Intersectionality

Further research on stress, health, and intersectionality is also needed because stress among parents of children with mental health needs is often treated as a uniform caregiving burden, when in reality it likely arises from multiple, interacting sources. Some stress may stem from the child's clinical needs and unpredictability of care, while other stress may be driven by institutional barriers, stigma, financial strain, workplace inflexibility, or adversarial service systems. Without disentangling these sources, interventions risk targeting symptoms rather than root causes.

Intersectional approaches are essential to this work because caregiving does not occur in a social vacuum. Parents occupy multiple social positions simultaneously, and these positions shape exposure to discrimination, access to accommodations, financial flexibility, and support networks. Treating caregiving stress as a singular experience obscures heterogeneity and may inadvertently center the experiences of more privileged families. An intersectional lens allows researchers to identify where stress is compounded by overlapping marginalization and where protective factors operate, providing a more precise foundation for designing equitable workplace, community, and policy interventions.

Policy Design and Usability

Next, there are many studies that have examined policy design and availability across differing political systems. However, there is a need to shift this inquiry from policy availability to policy usability as doing so asks a different yet critical set of questions. We know a great deal about whether paid leave exists, whether flexible work policies are on the books, and whether organizations formally endorse supervisor support. We know far less about whether parents of children with mental health disabilities can actually use these supports without cost, risk, or unintended consequences.

Another unresolved issue is disclosure. Many workplace supports require some explanation of need, even when policies are framed as universal. We do not yet understand which policy designs truly minimize disclosure and whether "minimal disclosure" models actually reduce stigma or simply shift scrutiny to performance metrics. For parents managing child mental health conditions, unpredictability complicates this further. We do not know which flexibility structures accommodate intermittent crises versus ongoing reduced capacity, and which models inadvertently increase workload for coworkers, thereby generating resentment and secondary stigma.

There is also limited knowledge about the interaction between formal policy and informal norms. Supervisor attitudes, team cultures, and workload redistribution practices often determine whether policies function as intended. Research on Family Supportive Supervisor Behaviors (Hammer et al., 2024) demonstrates that supervisors can be trained to provide emotional and instrumental support, model balance, and creatively manage work demands, with measurable reductions in work–family conflict. However, most of this evidence is drawn from general employee populations and does not isolate the experiences of parents caring for children with disabilities or mental health needs. We do not yet know whether this group requires a distinct configuration of supervisory practices, for example, greater emphasis on crisis responsiveness, confidentiality protections, or workload buffering mechanisms. Nor do we know whether standard supportive behaviors are sufficient when caregiving demands are unpredictable and stigmatized. Future research should therefore examine whether disability-related caregiving contexts call for tailored supervisory competencies beyond those identified in existing work–family intervention models.

Similarly, there is limited evidence on what actually happens to team workloads when a caregiver uses flexible arrangements, such as reduced hours or schedule adjustments. It is unclear whether tasks are redistributed equitably, absorbed informally by coworkers, or deferred in ways that increase strain elsewhere. Without understanding these dynamics, flexibility policies may unintentionally generate perceptions of unfairness or resentment that undermine team cohesion and stigma reduction efforts.

From an implementation perspective, we do not yet understand why some organizations achieve sustained exceptional caregiver retention while others do not, even when policies look similar on paper. Experimental and quasi-experimental studies could test specific features such as default flexibility options, anonymous request systems, protected scheduling blocks, or universal caregiver leave banks. Realist evaluation approaches could examine for whom these features work, in what contexts, and through which mechanisms. For example, does predictable scheduling reduce stress primarily by increasing perceived control, by improving childcare coordination, or by reducing conflict with supervisors? Identifying mechanisms would allow more precise intervention design.

Finally, we know relatively little about the long-term consequences of usable work–family policy for employees who provide exceptional care to a child with a mental health disability. Although flexibility, supervisor support, and schedule control are associated with reduced work–family conflict and improved well-being in general employee samples, most studies rely on cross-sectional or short-term designs and rarely disaggregate caregivers facing high-intensity, unpredictable demands. Research suggests that flexible arrangements may reduce immediate strain while producing ambiguous or even negative implications for advancement and earnings depending on context, yet these analyses seldom examine families managing chronic, stigmatized care needs. Even intervention studies that show improvements in sleep and stress biomarkers over 12 months do not tell us whether such gains translate into sustained workforce participation, cumulative reductions in stress exposure, or improved family functioning over years among disability caregiving families. Without longitudinal and mixed methods research centered on parents of children with mental health disabilities, we cannot determine whether usable policy produces durable structural inclusion for these families or merely delays workforce exit under conditions of escalating care demands.

Intervention Research and Evidence Gaps

In addition to descriptive and explanatory gaps, there is a striking lack of intervention research focused on families of children with mental health needs in work contexts. Very few studies have rigorously examined interventions designed to support parents in navigating disclosure, flexibility, and care coordination, or to shift organizational practices in ways that reduce stigma and risk for caregivers. Existing intervention-oriented work remains fragmented and underutilized in the broader work family and mental health literatures. Preliminary evidence from pilot intervention studies (Stewart et al., under review), on workplace disclosure decision support for parents of children with mental health needs, demonstrates both feasibility and strong demand for structured, evidence-informed tools that help families navigate complex employment decisions. Earlier intervention research by Stewart et al. (2022) on training human resources professionals highlights the potential for organizational-level capacity building to improve responses to employees with caregiving responsibilities, yet this line of work has not been systematically extended or replicated.

Classic contributions by Gates (2000) underscore the importance of employer-based interventions and internal organizational change strategies, particularly those that focus on supervisor education, policy translation, and workplace culture. However, much of this work predates contemporary labor market conditions, current mental health prevalence patterns, and evolving models of flexible work. Future research should prioritize the development, testing, and scaling of interventions at multiple levels, including family-facing decision aids, supervisor and HR training models, and organizational policy implementation strategies. Mixed methods trials, hybrid effectiveness implementation designs, and participatory approaches are especially well suited to advancing this agenda and ensuring that interventions are responsive to real-world family needs and organizational constraints.

Implications for Intervention and Translation to Practice

Finally, research should prioritize translation into practice. This includes developing and testing decision aids, supervisor training models, and organizational interventions that reflect real-world family dynamics and longitudinal care trajectories. Partnering with families, employers, and community organizations will be critical to ensuring that future research produces actionable knowledge capable of informing policy reform and workplace change.

Part 5: Conclusion

Uncertainty remains an enduring feature of exceptional caregiving, particularly for families raising children with mental health disabilities. Yet within a social work framework, uncertainty is not solely an individual burden to be endured in isolation. Across the chapters of this book, parents emerge not as passive recipients of services, but as skilled decision-makers operating within complex person-in-environment systems. They continuously assess risk, weigh competing obligations, and make strategic choices across family, work, school, and community contexts. Their actions reflect core social work competencies of assessment, critical thinking, and ethical decision-making under conditions of constrained resources and uneven institutional support.

The challenge before us is not to eliminate uncertainty, which is neither realistic nor desirable in dynamic family systems, but to redistribute responsibility for managing it. Social work's commitment to dignity and worth of the person and to social justice requires that we move beyond individual coping narratives toward structural accountability. Systems must recognize fluctuating caregiving demands, reduce punitive consequences when families seek accommodation, and design policies that protect rather than penalize those navigating the exceptional care related to caring for a child with a disability.

Supporting parents of children with mental health disabilities demands that we fully engage the person-in-environment perspective. Caregivers' decisions are shaped not only by individual resilience, but by workplace cultures, service availability, insurance structures, educational systems, and stigma embedded in public discourse. Competent practice therefore requires attention to micro-level engagement, mezzo-level organizational change, and macro-level policy advocacy. Decision-making processes themselves must be valued as sites of intervention, not merely as precursors to outcomes.

As scholars, practitioners, policymakers, and employers, we are called to build infrastructures of care that accompany families through uncertainty. This includes creating safe disclosure pathways in workplaces, embedding decision supports in service systems, and advancing policies that align with lived caregiving realities. In doing so, we affirm that navigating the unknown is not simply a personal journey, but a collective ethical obligation grounded in the core values and competencies of social work practice.

References

Blom, R., Jaspers, E., Knies, E., & van der Lippe, T. (2025). Family-friendly policies and workplace supports: A meta-analysis of their effects on career, job, and work-family outcomes. *Journal of Vocational Behavior*, *157*, 104091. https://doi.org/10.1016/j.jvb.2025.104091

Gates, L. B. (2000). Workplace accommodation as a social process. *Journal of Occupational Rehabilitation*, *10*(1), 85–98. https://doi.org/10.1023/A:1009445929841

Geraldes, D., Chambel, M. J., & Carvalho, V. S. (2024). Supervisor support and work-family practices: A systematic review. *Societies*, *14*(12), 272. https://doi.org/10.3390/soc14120272

Gray, D. E. (2002). Everybody just freezes. Everybody is just embarrassed: Felt and enacted stigma among parents of children with high functioning autism. *Sociology of Health & Illness*, *24*(6), 734–749. https://doi.org/10.1111/1467-9566.00316

Hammer, L. B., Dimoff, J., Mohr, C. D., & Allen, S. J. (2024). A framework for protecting and promoting employee mental health through supervisor supportive behaviors. *Occupational Health Science*, *8*, 243–268. https://doi.org/10.1007/s41542-023-00171-x

Kinnear, S. H., Link, B. G., Ballan, M. S., & Fischbach, R. L. (2016). Understanding the experience of stigma for parents of children with autism spectrum disorder and the role stigma plays in families' lives. *Journal of Autism and Developmental Disorders*, *46*(3), 942–953. https://doi.org/10.1007/s10803-015-2637-9

Leso, V., Carugno, M., Carrer, P., Fusco, F., Mendola, M., Coppola, M., Zaffina, S., Di Prinzio, R. R., & Iavicoli, I. (2024). The Total Worker Health® (TWH) approach: A systematic review of its application in different occupational settings. *BMC Public Health*, *24*(1), 2037. https://doi.org/10.1186/s12889-024-19500-y

National Institute for Occupational Safety and Health. (2016). *Fundamentals of Total Worker Health® approaches: Essential elements for advancing worker safety, health, and well-being* (NIOSH Publication No. 2017-112). Centers for Disease Control and Prevention. https://www.cdc.gov/niosh/docs/2017-112/

National Institute for Occupational Safety and Health. (2024). *What Is Total Worker Health?* Centers for Disease Control and Prevention. https://www.cdc.gov/niosh/twh/overview.html

Rosenzweig, J. M., Barnett, R. C., Huffstutter, K., & Stewart, L. M. (2008). Work-life integration: History, theory and strategy. In J. M. Rosenzweig & E. M. Brennan (Eds.), *Work, life, and the mental health system of care: A guide for professionals supporting families of children with emotional or behavioral disorders* (pp. 89–115). Paul H. Brookes.

Rosenzweig, J. M., Huffstutter, K., Malsch, A., Stewart, L. M. & Brennan, E. M. (2011). Voices at the table: Views of parents and human resource professionals on managing the work-family boundary. *Special Issue on Family Voices/Perspectives for Best Practices in Mental Health: An International Journal*, *7*(1), 67–93.

Sellmaier, C., & Buckingham, S. (2022). "I think sometimes that dads are kind of forgotten (…) so it's nice that we also get a voice.": Work-life experiences of employed U.S. fathers caring for a child with special health care needs. *Community, Work, & Family*, *25*(5), 661–676. https://doi.org/10.1080/13668803.2021.1911935

Sellmaier, C., Stewart, L. M., & Brennan, E. M. (2020). Workforce engagement of parents of children and youth with mental health difficulties: The impact of community services and supports. *Community Work & Family*, *23*(5), 534–555. https://doi.org/10.1080/13668803.2020.1820954

Stewart, L. M. (2013). Family care responsibilities and employment: Exploring the impact of type of family care on work–family and family–work conflict. *Journal of Family Issues*, *34*(7), 873–896. https://doi.org/10.1177/0192513X12437708

Stewart, L. M., & Charles, A. (2022). To disclose or conceal? Workplace disability and eldercare-related disclosure decision-making strategies. *Journal of Family Issues*, *43*(6), 1536–1554. https://doi.org/10.1177/0192513X211026965

Stewart, L. M., Rosenzweig, J. M., Malsch Tamarkin, A. M., Brennan, E. M., & Lukefahr, J. (2022). Expanding workplace inclusion of employees who are parents of children with disabilities through diversity training. *Healthcare*, *10*(12), 2361. https://doi.org/10.3390/healthcare10122361

Stewart, L. M., Sellmaier, C., Brannan, A. M., & Brennan, E. M. (2023). Family demands and workplace supports of employed parents of children with typical and exceptional care responsibilities and their effects on conflict and stress. *Journal of Child and Family Studies*, *32*(4), 1048–1064. https://doi.org/10.1007/s10826-022-02363-5

Stewart, **L.M.**, Sellmaier, C., Cossio, M., & Morales, M. (under review). Pilot of a Workplace Disclosure Decision Aid and Resources for Employed Parents.

Stewart, L. M., Sellmaier, C., Henderson-Posther, M., Lukefahr, J., & Brennan, E. M. (2025). Navigating stigma and discrimination at work while parenting a child with a mental health disability. In P. N. Claster & S. L. Blair (Eds.), *Disability and the family: Challenges, resources, and resilience* (Vol. 27, p. 0). Emerald Publishing Limited. https://doi.org/10.1108/S1530-353520250000027005

Stewart, L. M., Stutz, H., & Lile, W. (2018). The continuum of dependent family care: A theoretical explanation and model. *Community, Work & Family*, *21*(5), 599–619. https://doi.org/10.1080/13668803.2018.1530637

U.S. Department of Education, Office for Civil Rights. (2023, November). *2020–21 Civil Rights Data Collection: Student discipline and school climate in U.S. public schools*. https://civilrightsdata.ed.gov/

GLOSSARY

Ableism A system of beliefs, practices, and institutional structures that privilege non-disabled norms and disadvantage individuals with disabilities and their families. *See also:* Structural stigma; Social model of disability.

Ambiguous loss A form of loss in which a person is physically present but psychologically changed, creating ongoing uncertainty and unresolved grief within families.

Behavioral Health Workforce Education and Training (WET) State-administered programs that support supervision capacity, training site development, and workforce pipeline expansion in behavioral health, particularly in underserved communities.

Boundary permeability The degree to which responsibilities and emotions from one life domain, such as work or family, cross into another. *See also:* Work–family fit; Work–family misfit.

Care continuum The range of caregiving demands, from typical parenting responsibilities to intensive, long-term support associated with disability or chronic conditions.

Caregiver strain The emotional, physical, relational, and economic stress experienced by individuals providing ongoing care. *See also:* Role strain.

Care intensity The level of time, coordination, supervision, and emotional labor required to meet caregiving responsibilities.

Care-related employment disruption Interruptions, reductions, or instability in employment resulting from caregiving demands associated with a child's mental health disability. *See also:* Work–family misfit; Crisis-driven caregiving.

Community–work–family interface The interaction among caregiving responsibilities, employment structures, and community systems that shapes family well-being and decision-making. *See also:* Person-in-environment.

Conservation of resources theory A theory of stress suggesting that individuals experience strain when valued resources—such as time, income, or social support—are threatened or depleted.

Continuum of dependent care A framework describing caregiving needs as existing along a continuum. Position along the continuum dictates care demands and resources. *See also:* Care continuum; Care intensity.

Council on Social Work Education (CSWE) The Council on Social Work Education is the accrediting body for graduate and undergraduate social work programs in the United States.

Courtesy stigma Negative judgments or discrimination directed toward individuals because of their association with a stigmatized person. *See also:* Structural stigma.

Crisis-driven caregiving Caregiving organized around unpredictable or acute episodes that disrupt routines and require rapid adaptation across systems.

Decision support (structured decision support) A systematic approach that provides information, value clarification tools, and communication strategies to support complex decision-making under uncertainty. In this book, structured decision support refers to tools assisting parents navigating workplace disclosure and caregiving decisions.

Decommodification The extent to which individuals can maintain well-being independent of labor market participation, often shaped by social policy.

Diagnostic gatekeeping The use of formal diagnostic criteria as thresholds for accessing services, accommodations, or institutional supports.

Disability A condition arising from the interaction between individual impairments and environmental, social, and institutional barriers that limit participation.

Disability justice An intersectional framework that centers collective access, leadership of those most impacted, and structural transformation of ableist systems. *See also:* Social model of disability.

Ecological fit The degree of alignment between family needs and the expectations, resources, and constraints of surrounding systems. *See also:* Person-in-environment.

Educational Policy and Accreditation Standards The Council on Social Work Education uses a competency-based framework to accredit social work programs in the United States. This framework consists of nine competencies, and the curriculum of accredited social work programs is oriented around these nine competencies.

Exceptional care responsibilities Intensive and sustained caregiving tasks that exceed normative parenting expectations and require ongoing coordination across systems.

Family resilience The capacity of families to adapt, reorganize, and maintain functioning in the face of stress or adversity.

Flexibility stigma Negative judgments or career penalties experienced by employees who use workplace flexibility for caregiving. *See also:* Ideal worker norm.

Ideal worker norm The expectation that workers prioritize employment above personal responsibilities and remain continuously available and unencumbered by caregiving demands.

Individuals with Disabilities Education Act (IDEA) U.S. federal legislation guaranteeing free and appropriate public education for eligible children with disabilities in the least restrictive environment.

Infrastructure of care The formal and informal systems, policies, and supports that enable families to manage caregiving responsibilities without disproportionate harm to economic stability or well-being.

Interdisciplinary training model An educational structure that integrates multiple professional disciplines in preparing practitioners to address complex social and health needs.

Life course theory A framework emphasizing how social, economic, and historical contexts shape individual and family trajectories over time.

Medical model of disability An approach that locates disability primarily within individual impairment and prioritizes diagnosis and treatment.

Mental health disability A condition involving emotional, behavioral, or psychological challenges that substantially affect functioning across life domains.

Navigating uncertainty The ongoing process through which caregivers assess fluctuating risks, resources, and institutional constraints while making decisions across work, family, and community domains.

Person-in-environment A foundational social work perspective that understands individuals within interacting social, institutional, economic, and cultural systems.

Prevalence The proportion of a population experiencing a particular condition within a specified period.

Respite care Temporary caregiving support designed to provide relief to primary caregivers.

Role strain Stress arising from incompatible or competing expectations across multiple social roles.

Section 504 U.S. civil rights legislation prohibiting discrimination against individuals with disabilities in federally funded programs.

Social justice A core social work value emphasizing equitable access to resources, opportunities, and protections for marginalized individuals and families.

Social model of disability A framework that locates disability in environmental and structural barriers rather than solely in individual impairment.

Spillover (positive and negative) The transfer of emotions, stress, or benefits from one life domain, such as work or family, into another.

Structural competency A practice framework emphasizing recognition of structural factors, such as policy and institutional design, that shape caregiving experiences.

Structural stigma Institutional policies and cultural norms that systematically disadvantage stigmatized groups.

Time bind The experience of insufficient time resulting from competing work and caregiving demands. Key proposition of role theory.

Work–family fit The degree of compatibility between employment structures and caregiving responsibilities.

Work–family misfit Persistent misalignment between caregiving demands and workplace expectations.

Work–life integration An approach that emphasizes blending or coordinating work and personal responsibilities rather than a focus on balancing them.

Workplace Disclosure The process by which individuals decide whether, when, and how to share information about disability-related needs within employment settings.

INDEX

For Product Safety Concerns and Information please contact our EU representative GPSR@taylorandfrancis.com
Taylor & Francis Verlag GmbH, Kaufingerstraße 24, 80331 München, Germany

www.ingramcontent.com/pod-product-compliance
Ingram Content Group UK Ltd.
Pitfield, Milton Keynes, MK11 3LW, UK
UKHW020009200926
475702UK00015B/2554
9781032847375